UNLOCKING ENERGY HEALTH

Discover the Surprising Role of Metabolism in Preventing Disease & Living a Life Full of Vitality

<u>CONRAD FORSYTHE</u>

Table of Contents

INTRODUCTION

The Power of Metabolism

A lot of people have a misunderstanding of metabolism because it's simplified to terms like "burning calories" & "weight loss." But there's more to it than that; it's a dynamic, intricate process that drives every physical component of our bodies. Metabolic processes impact every aspect of living things, including energy production, immune system defense, brain function, & daily resilience. When our metabolism is in top shape, we have boundless energy, sharp minds, & solid health as a whole. Our energy drops & our susceptibility to exhaustion, brain fog, & illness increases when it's out of whack, which can happen as a result of stress, inactivity, or bad nutrition.

Discover the surprising & crucial role of metabolism in enabling us to live a resilient & energetic life in Unlocking Energy Health. By delving into the inner workings of your body's energy production system, you will learn how to achieve & maintain optimal health, rather than relying on superficial health trends. In this course, you will gain knowledge about the science behind energy health & how metabolic flexibility, or the body's capacity to switch between energy sources, can aid in maintaining strength, energy, & adaptability in the face of life's challenges.

Join me as we delve into the fundamentals of metabolism: its nature, its cellular mechanisms, & the universal relevance of this knowledge across all age groups. After that, we'll examine how your energy & health are affected by the four main components of metabolic health: food, exercise, sleep, & stress management. Gaining knowledge of how to fuel & maintain your metabolism will equip you with the means to sustain long-term energy, mental clarity, & resilience to chronic diseases.

Learn how to optimize your metabolism & live a vital, healthy life with the help of this book's thorough, science-based approach & practical strategies. Each chapter includes actionable steps to help you put what you learn into practice, including nutrition, meal timing, exercise, & restorative practices. Additionally, we will go over the ways in which metabolism changes with age, providing you with tools to help your metabolism thrive at every stage of life.

In addition to providing information on how to speed up your metabolism, Unlocking Energy Health extends an invitation to adopt a way of life that boosts stamina, vitality, & health. Managing your energy levels, lowering your risk of disease, & improving your quality of life can all be achieved by learning about & taking care of your metabolism. Come with me as we delve into the vast possibilities of energy health & discover how to live each day to the fullest, fueled by a sense of empowerment & vitality.

Understanding Metabolism & Energy Health

Many people compare metabolism to the body's engine because of the intricate web of chemical reactions that it employs to transform the fuel our cells require—oxygen & the food we consume—into usable energy. The most visible processes, like movement & brain activity, rely on this energy, while the most subtle processes, like cellular repair, hormone regulation, & immune response, are also dependent on it. Metabolic breakdown, or catabolism, releases energy by breaking down molecules, & anabolism, or the building up of the body through the utilization of this energy, are the two basic processes that make up metabolism. This intricate equilibrium is fundamental for maintaining life, & by comprehending its operation, we can maximize the body's capacity for vitality, health, & longevity.

Metabolism revolves around the notion of energy health, which extends beyond the simple act of "burning calories." A state of energy health is one in which one's bodily systems are able to generate & utilize energy in an optimal manner, allowing one to carry out all physiological functions with vigor & health. Metabolic flexibility, the ability to use various fuel sources (carbs & fats, for example) in response to changes in supply & demand, is required for this. Both adjusting to new forms of physical activity & keeping one's energy levels consistent throughout the day depend on metabolic flexibility. Better health outcomes & a decreased risk of chronic diseases like diabetes & cardiovascular disorders are achieved when our metabolism is flexible & adaptable, allowing us to easily handle changes in our environment, diet, & lifestyle.

The mitochondria, sometimes referred to as the "powerhouse" of the cell, play an important role in metabolic processes. Mitochondria are small cellular organelles that play a key role in cellular energy storage & transfer by converting food into adenosine triphosphate (ATP). Optimal mitochondrial function is essential for metabolic health because it allows for efficient energy production, reduces oxidative stress, & aids in cellular health maintenance. Fatigue, inefficient energy production, & an increased risk of metabolic diseases can result from impaired mitochondrial function, which can be caused by aging, stress, an unhealthy diet, & an inactive lifestyle. As a result, preserving metabolic health as a whole requires safeguarding & promoting mitochondrial health via dietary, exercise, & lifestyle choices.

A person's diet has a significant impact on their metabolic rate. Metabolism is a process by which the three main dietary macronutrients—carbohydrates, lipids, & proteins—influence energy production & metabolic health in their own distinct ways. Fats supply a more sustained energy reserve that can be utilized when glucose levels are low, while carbohydrates are usually broken down into glucose, the body's preferred quick-energy source. Comparatively, proteins are mainly involved in tissue repair & construction but can also be converted into energy when necessary. To make dietary choices that support optimal metabolic function, it is helpful to understand how these macronutrients impact energy production. Additionally, the body's capacity to generate energy & sustain metabolic health is aided by specific micronutrients & vitamins, including coenzyme Q10, magnesium, & B vitamins, which have vital functions in metabolic pathways.

In addition to a healthy diet, regular physical activity is essential for a healthy metabolism. When you work out, your body demands more energy, so it adjusts its metabolism to be more efficient & flexible. This is particularly true for activities that test your cardiovascular endurance & muscular strength. When it comes to improving mitochondrial function & increasing metabolic rate, even when at rest, high-intensity interval training (HIIT) & resistance training really shine. Strength training like this increases the body's mitochondrial biogenesis, or its ability to generate energy. To keep blood sugar levels steady & ward off metabolic diseases like diabetes, regular exercise helps increase insulin sensitivity.

Metabolic wellness also requires proper sleep & stress management. During a good night's sleep, the body repairs damaged cells, regulates hormones, & consolidates memories. Metabolic dysregulation, increased hunger, & decreased insulin sensitivity are all consequences of these processes being disturbed by inadequate or poor sleep. However, cortisol is a hormone that can negatively impact metabolic health when elevated for long periods of time; it promotes fat storage, increases blood sugar levels, & decreases muscle mass. This is in contrast to the beneficial effects of short-term stress. Keeping cortisol levels in check & supporting metabolic balance can be achieved through stress management practices such as mindfulness, meditation, & regular physical activity.

An integrative perspective on energy utilization & regulation is necessary for a complete comprehension of metabolic health & energy balance. Producing an internal environment that supports resilience, adaptability, & energy production is more important than calorie intake versus calorie expenditure. We can improve our metabolic health &, by implication, our quality of life, by eating nutrient-dense foods, exercising regularly, getting enough restful sleep, & dealing with stress. We can enhance our daily energy levels, protect ourselves from chronic diseases, support mental clarity, & cultivate a sense of vitality & well-being throughout life by making informed lifestyle choices based on this foundational knowledge of metabolism.

What is Metabolism?

All the chemical reactions that the body does to sustain life & function are collectively known as metabolism. In addition to providing energy to every cell in our body, this intricate & well-coordinated mechanism keeps our internal balance, or homeostasis, so that we can respond appropriately to the many demands & stresses that we encounter on a daily basis. Metabolic process is fundamental because it transforms oxygen & food into energy that drives all of our bodily functions, from breathing to thinking to the most minute, invisible cellular operations. The complex system is always at action, with the two main components being anabolism & catabolism. Metabolic breakdown produces energy, whereas anabolism constructs & synthesizes molecules to sustain development, repair, & cellular structure. When together, these mechanisms keep the fragile equilibrium necessary for life to persist. A thorough understanding of metabolism requires dissecting it into its component parts & seeing how they all work together to promote energy health & ward against sickness.

Metabolic rate, the rate at which certain chemical reactions take place in the organism, is the primary idea in metabolism. Factors including heredity, age, body type, &

way of life all contribute to an individual's metabolic rate. A person's energy levels, weight, & stress tolerance can all be impacted by their metabolic rate, which is a measure of how effectively energy is burned. The opposite is true for those with a low metabolic rate; this conserves energy inside the body, which might make them feel lethargic, gain weight, or experience weariness. At rest, the body uses the very minimum of energy—its basal metabolic rate—to keep vital organs like the heart, lungs, & temperature stable. Body mass index (BMI) differs greatly from one individual to the next yet makes up a significant amount of daily calorie expenditure. To harness or improve metabolism through dietary changes, exercise, & stress management, it is helpful to understand one's metabolic rate & the variables that can affect it.

The mitochondria are little organelles inside our cells that are responsible for converting food into adenosine triphosphate (ATP), the molecule that provides energy for almost every process in the body. The effectiveness of mitochondria has a direct impact on the amount of energy that can be used for daily activities, cognitive function, & physical activity; thus, mitochondria are fundamental to metabolic health. The mitochondria are engaged in a wide variety of cellular processes, including energy production, signal transduction, growth, & programmed cell death (apoptosis). If mitochondria are healthy, the metabolism is robust; if they are damaged, the metabolism slows, oxidative stress rises, & metabolic illnesses are more likely to occur. Proper nutrition, frequent exercise, & reducing exposure to pollutants are habits that maintain mitochondrial health, since mitochondrial activity can decline with age or as a result of lifestyle-related pressures.

Another crucial part of comprehending metabolism is the idea of metabolic flexibility. The capacity to efficiently transition between various energy sources, such glucose & fat, in response to the availability & demand of these resources is known as metabolic flexibility. Promoting stability in blood sugar levels, decreasing hunger fluctuations, & delivering sustained energy throughout the day, a flexible metabolism is better equipped to adjust to changes in nutrition, physical activity, & other environmental influences. people who are metabolically flexible are better able to manage fasting or periods of intense activity without suffering from severe energy crashes; on the other hand, people who are metabolically rigid may have problems controlling their weight, dealing with blood sugar imbalances, or both. The foundation of resilient & long-lasting energy health is metabolic flexibility, which can be achieved by a combination of different types of exercise (aerobic, anaerobic, & resistance training), as well as certain dietary patterns (such as balanced macronutrient consumption or intermittent fasting).

The body uses certain nutrients to power metabolic pathways & cellular functions, therefore proper nutrition is essential for sustaining metabolism. Different from one another, carbohydrates, proteins, & lipids all have a role in generating energy. For example, during physical exertion, the brain & muscles rely on glucose, a fuel that is quickly produced after carbohydrate digestion. Hormone synthesis & cellular structure rely on stored fats, which also serve as a more stable energy source. Proteins can be turned into energy when needed, in addition to their primary usage in tissue repair & construction. In addition to these macronutrients, micronutrients like minerals & vitamins are essential for a number of metabolic processes. To give only a few examples, the B vitamins are involved in energy production as coenzymes, magnesium is crucial for ATP synthesis, & iron is involved in cellular respiration & oxygen transport. The foundation for a healthy metabolism is a diet that is both balanced & full of complete foods.

A person's level of physical activity is an important factor in their metabolic health. Exercising, particularly in ways that test the heart & muscles, triggers mechanisms that improve metabolism on a molecular level. The increased need for energy during exercise trains the body to produce ATP more efficiently. Researchers have discovered that regular exercise, especially HIIT & resistance training, raises the number of mitochondria in muscle cells, which in turn increases their ability to produce energy & their metabolic rate, even when at rest. As an added bonus, regular exercise increases insulin sensitivity, a key factor in preventing metabolic diseases like type 2 diabetes by keeping blood sugar levels steady. Incorporating a range of physical activities into one's routine can help improve energy wellness in the long run by increasing metabolic rate & metabolic flexibility.

The effects of stress & sleep are another critical component of metabolic health. The body repairs damaged cells, regulates hormones, & consolidates memories during quality sleep, among many other metabolic functions. Metabolic dysregulation, increased hunger, & decreased insulin sensitivity are all brought on by a lack of or poor quality sleep, which interrupts these processes. Similarly, metabolism can be negatively impacted by chronic stress. The stress hormone cortisol is responsible for the accumulation of fat, the atrophy of muscular tissue, & the disruption of normal blood sugar levels; in the long run, it can damage metabolic function. Metabolic function can be supported by stress management practices including mindfulness, meditation, & physical activity, as well as by making restorative sleep a priority. These practices assist the body maintain energy balance & reduce the detrimental effects of stress hormones.

All things considered, the metabolic process is a complex web that controls the conversion & utilization of energy within our bodies. Genetics, way of life, environment, & mental health are just a few of the many aspects that might impact it. If we want to improve our health, have more energy, & feel more vital, we need to learn what metabolism is & how to support it. Metabolism is more accurately understood as a dynamic system that changes in response to our lifestyle choices, including food, exercise, & stress management, than as a fixed attribute or a process limited to burning calories. Informed lifestyle choices that promote metabolic health can improve our physical, mental, & emotional health, laying the groundwork for a long, healthy, & vibrant life.

Breaking Down Metabolism

Fueling every bodily function, from repairing cells to regulating hormones, metabolism is the complex process by which the body turns food & oxygen into energy. Rather than being a singular process, it is really a web of interdependent chemical reactions that convert the food we eat into energy. Catabolism involves the breakdown of molecules to release energy, while anabolism involves the use of that energy to construct & repair tissues. These reactions can be broadly categorized into two main processes. Catabolism supplies the energy required for anabolism, ensuring that these processes are constantly balanced. When combined, they create a cycle that gives life-sustaining energy & keeps everything in its proper equilibrium.

Metabolic function relies heavily on cellular components, most notably mitochondria, the so-called "powerhouses" of the cell. Adenosine triphosphate (ATP) is the molecule that stores energy for cellular functions. These small organelles convert nutrients, particularly glucose & fatty acids, into ATP. ATP is like a "energy currency," giving cells the power they need right when they need it. Optimal metabolism relies on mitochondrial efficiency for energy production, oxidative stress mitigation, & cellular health maintenance. But mitochondrial health—& metabolic efficiency—can be affected by things like age, food, & lifestyle. We can promote metabolic health & sustained energy levels over time by learning about mitochondrial health & supporting it through healthy eating, regular exercise, & other lifestyle choices.

The pace at which the body converts energy is known as metabolic rate, & it is an important part of metabolism. When at rest, the body requires a certain amount of energy—its basal metabolic rate, or BMR—to keep essential processes running smoothly, like breathing, blood circulation, & temperature regulation. Our ability to burn calories & keep energy levels up is impacted by a number of factors, including our metabolic rate, which is in turn influenced by things like age, genetics, body composition, & physical activity. Those whose metabolic rates are higher are more likely to burn calories quickly & have an easier time keeping their weight steady, while those whose rates are lower may have more trouble conserving energy & controlling their weight. Exercises that increase muscular mass, mitochondrial density, & metabolic flexibility, such as high-intensity interval training (HIIT) & resistance training, are known to increase metabolic rate.

Metabolic flexibility refers to the capacity of the body to utilize various fuel sources, like carbohydrates & fats, in response to energy demands & availability. Maintaining steady blood sugar levels & minimal energy swings are hallmarks of a metabolically flexible system, which allows the body to effectively adjust to changes in food, exercise, & energy demands. People whose metabolic flexibility is impaired may find it difficult to control their weight, feel constantly hungry, or both. Better regulation of energy production & storage can be achieved through improved metabolic flexibility, which can be achieved through specific dietary & lifestyle practices like a varied exercise regimen, intermittent fasting, & a balanced intake of macronutrients.

The metabolism depends on nutrition because different metabolic pathways are powered by different nutrients. Different from one another, carbohydrates, proteins, & fats all play a role in generating energy. For low-intensity, sustained activities, carbohydrates are ideal because they are rapidly converted into glucose, which provides energy right away, while fats provide a longer-lasting reserve. Proteins are mainly involved in repairing damaged tissues, but they can also be converted into energy if needed. Micronutrients, such as iron, magnesium, & the B vitamins, are just as important as macronutrients when it comes to metabolic processes, supporting cellular respiration & functioning as coenzymes. To keep metabolism running smoothly, one must consume a nutrient-dense diet that is abundant in minerals & vitamins.

A healthy metabolism is dependent on more than just food & exercise. During sleep, the body repairs itself, controls hormone levels, & strengthens memories. A disruption in metabolic regulation, an increase in hunger, & a decrease in insulin sensitivity can result from chronic sleep deprivation. Chronic stress raises cortisol levels, which can hinder metabolism by encouraging fat storage, raising blood sugar levels, & decreasing muscle mass; thus, stress management is equally important. To keep your metabolism in check & protect it from cortisol's harmful effects on your energy processes, make getting enough sleep a priority & learn to manage stress through mindfulness & exercise.

To understand metabolism in its entirety, one must acknowledge it as an adaptive system that is constantly changing in response to both internal & external stimuli. Diet, exercise, mental health, & environmental factors all have an impact on this responsive process, rather than a static attribute. One way to improve one's physical energy, health, mental resilience, & overall vitality is to gain a better understanding of metabolism & how to support it through mindful lifestyle choices. Promoting metabolic health is a self-determinative strategy for health & wellness that can improve life quality across the lifespan by providing the fuel for an active, healthy lifestyle.

Metabolic Rate: The Basics

A person's metabolic rate—the pace at which their body uses energy to maintain essential bodily functions—is an important factor in their general well-being, energy levels, & ability to control their weight. The efficiency with which the body converts food into energy is fundamentally influenced by metabolic rate. This energy is subsequently utilized for numerous processes, including respiration, blood circulation, cell growth & repair, & temperature regulation. An individual's basal metabolic rate (BMR) is the sum of all the calories required to maintain metabolic function when the body is at rest & not actively working out. The basal metabolic rate (BMR) is the most important component of total daily energy expenditure; it can vary greatly from one person to another & can make up as much as 60–75% of it. Age, gender, genetics, hormonal regulation, body composition, & genetics are some of the factors that impact basal metabolic rate (BMR). People who are physically fit tend to have a higher basal metabolic rate (BMR) because their muscles use more energy during exercise than their fat cells. A person's metabolic rate naturally drops after the age of 30, due to the loss of muscle mass & the onset of hormonal changes, so age is another important factor. The basal metabolic rate (BMR) is different for men & women because men typically have a larger percentage of muscle mass. These differences highlight the fact that metabolic rate is very individual, affected by a combination of genetics & environmental factors. Understanding the function of mitochondria is essential for comprehending energy production, as it is a key component of metabolism that has a direct effect on metabolic rate. In order to generate energy, the body must first convert nutrients into adenosine triphosphate (ATP). This process is carried out by mitochondria, which are organelles found within cells. The overall metabolic rate is heavily dependent on how efficiently mitochondria function; a higher metabolic rate & better energy levels are the result of optimal mitochondrial function, which allows for more efficient production of energy. On the flip side, malfunctioning mitochondria can reduce energy production, which in turn causes metabolic disorders, fatigue, & weight gain. Hence, a healthy metabolic rate requires supporting mitochondrial health via good nutrition, frequent exercise, & stress management. Resting metabolic rate (RMR) is an additional important component of metabolic rate; it is comparable to basal metabolic rate (BMR) but is measured under somewhat different circumstances. Unlike basal metabolic rate (BMR), which can only be calculated under specific conditions (i.e., while fasting & after a full night's sleep), resting metabolic rate (RMR) can be measured at any time of day & is affected by a wider range of variables, such as levels of physical activity, stress, & recent dietary consumption. Although RMR & BMR are closely related, RMR is usually slightly higher. Having a good grasp of RMR can empower individuals to more accurately assess their daily energy requirements, leading to more tailored approaches to weight management & general well-being. Aside from basal metabolic rate (BMR) & resting metabolic rate (RMR), two additional factors that impact total metabolic rate are the thermic effect of food (TEF) & the thermic effect of exercise (TEE). How much energy is needed for food digestion, absorption, & processing is called total energetic expenditure (TEF). Protein, in particular, has a greater thermic effect than carbs or fats, so consuming meals high in protein can marginally increase metabolism during digestion. Contrarily, total energy expenditure (TEE) stands for the amount of energy that is used up when working out. Both the duration & intensity of physical activity, particularly strength training & HIIT, have been shown to considerably raise metabolic rate. What we call the "afterburn" effect or excess post-exercise oxygen consumption (EPOC) happens when your metabolism stays high for a while after a strenuous workout. This phenomenon exemplifies the positive effects of increased metabolic rates on active individuals who engage in regular exercise. A less well-known component of total metabolic rate is non-exercise activity thermogenesis (NEAT), which can occur even when no structured exercise is taking place. This includes things like fidgeting, walking, & using the stairs. Higher levels of NEAT are associated with better metabolic health, & it includes all forms of physical activity other than exercise. One important thing to remember is that metabolic rate is not a static but rather a complex system that can be affected by various factors both inside & outside of the body. Because of this adaptability, metabolic rate can be changed over time by making deliberate adjustments to one's way of life. One way to increase energy expenditure is to build muscle through resistance training. Another way is to modify one's diet to make it more metabolically efficient. Lastly, one can optimize their stress & sleep levels to further increase metabolic rate. Consistent effort can bring about metabolic adaptations like enhanced mitochondrial efficiency & metabolic flexibility, which in turn lead to long-term advantages in managing weight, preventing diseases, & feeling vital. The body can function at its metabolic peak when one prioritizes lifestyle factors that promote metabolic health, such as nutrient-dense food, enough water, enough sleep, & stress management. To further optimize metabolism & maintain steady energy production, nutrient timing is important. This includes making sure to consume protein first thing in the morning & eating balanced meals throughout the day. The metabolic rate also takes into account how the body adjusts to changes in caloric intake, whether from starvation or excessive eating. In an attempt to conserve energy, the body may lower the metabolic rate when people drastically cut back on their caloric intake. Adaptive thermogenesis is the process that makes it harder to lose weight over the long term when calorie restriction is done for an extended period of time. Overfeeding, on the other hand, can disrupt metabolism, which in turn can cause insulin resistance & fat storage. Achieving & maintaining a healthy weight requires a delicate balancing act between caloric intake & energy expenditure, as well as metabolic health. A person's metabolic rate is critically affected by their genes. A person's metabolic rate, or the rate at which their body processes nutrients, burns calories, & stores fat, is influenced by both hereditary factors & lifestyle choices. Although some people may be born with a faster metabolism than average, others may need to take more active steps to keep or speed up their metabolism if theirs is naturally slower. New insights into the effects of individual genetic variations on metabolic rate are emerging from genomic research, which may one day lead to more personalized recommendations for food & exercise. To sum up, metabolic rate is an essential component of health since it controls the body's energy generation efficiency across many different processes. Gaining control of your health can be as simple as learning your metabolic rate, which can lead to better weight management, more energy, & a decreased risk of metabolic diseases. Maintaining a high metabolic rate is the cornerstone of long-term health, so it's important to pay attention to things like muscle mass, mitochondrial health, exercise, nutrition, & sleep. If you want to feel better physically, have more stamina, & be less susceptible to illness, then you need to put in the work to keep up with this dynamic & responsive system.

Factors that Affect Metabolism

A complex web of internal & external influences affects metabolism, which in turn determines the body's energy processing & utilization efficiency. Heredity is one of the main determinants of metabolic rate. A person's metabolic rate is heavily influenced by their genetic composition, which in turn affects their basal metabolic rate (BMR), fat burning efficiency, & glucose processing efficiency. For instance, whereas some people may be born with a slower metabolism & so burn calories less efficiently, others may be born with a higher metabolism & thus burn calories more efficiently. Hormone control & mitochondrial function are two areas that can be impacted by these genetic variables, which in turn can impact energy expenditure & weight management. While heredity does provide the groundwork, environmental variables & lifestyle choices play much larger roles in regulating metabolic rate. Being physically active is one of the most important aspects of a healthy lifestyle. The metabolic rate is significantly impacted by exercise, especially resistance training & HIIT. On top of boosting calorie expenditure during exercise, regular physical activity also accelerates calorie burning after exercise, a phenomenon called excess post-exercise oxygen consumption (EPOC) or the afterburn effect. Boosting metabolic efficiency & encouraging fat reduction, this increased calorie burn can continue for hours after exercise. Plus, lifting weights increases muscular mass, which in turn increases the basal metabolic rate (BMR), which means you'll burn more calories over the long run compared to when you were adipose. This is because muscle tissue is more energy dense than fat tissue. One of the most important factors influencing metabolism is age. Loss of lean muscle mass & changes in hormone control are the main reasons why people's metabolic rates tend to decline as they age. The basal metabolic rate (BMR) starts to fall by about 1-2 percent every decade beyond the age of 30, which can cause weight gain if exercise & nutrition aren't changed accordingly. Anabolic hormone levels, including testosterone & growth hormone, which are involved in preserving muscle mass & metabolic function, decline with age, & this slowdown in metabolism is associated with that. Hormonal changes are just as important as muscle mass for controlling metabolism. Important hormones for metabolic regulation include leptin, insulin, thyroid hormone, cortisol, & thyroid hormone. As an example, hormones secreted by the thyroid gland govern the rate at which cells burn calories, thereby regulating the body's metabolism. A slowed metabolism, increased body fat, & lethargy are symptoms of hypothyroidism, a disorder in which the thyroid gland does not generate enough hormones. Conversely, symptoms such as anxiety & weight loss might result from an overactive metabolism caused by hyperthyroidism, a condition in which the thyroid generates an excess of hormone. Another hormone that has an immediate effect on metabolism is insulin, which controls blood sugar levels. Increased blood sugar levels & possible weight gain can occur as a result of insulin resistance, a disorder that is frequently associated with obesity & inactivity. Chronic stress can cause levels of the stress hormone cortisol to rise, which in turn encourages fat deposition, especially in the abdominal region, & worsens metabolic health. As a hormone that controls energy balance & hunger, leptin is also involved in metabolism; when levels are low, one tends to eat more & burn less fat. Metabolic rate is affected by dietary factors as well. The effectiveness of metabolism can be greatly affected by the kinds of food that are eaten. It takes more energy to digest, absorb, & metabolize protein-rich diets compared to carbs or lipids, for example, because of their higher thermic effect. A temporary rise in metabolic rate can be achieved by this enhanced energy expenditure. Green tea, chili peppers, & coffee are just a few foods that include components like capsaicin & catechins, which can give you a little metabolic boost. Conversely, metabolic dysfunction can result from a diet high in processed foods & refined sugars, which can increase inflammation & insulin resistance. By reducing the likelihood of sharp swings in blood sugar & energy levels, eating smaller, more often meals can also help maintain a steady metabolic rate. Crucial factors to consider, nevertheless, are calorie consumption & macronutrient balance. Gaining weight is possible with an excess of calories, even from nutritious foods, whereas a slowdown in metabolism due to energy conservation is the consequence of an inadequate calorie intake. A crucial but frequently disregarded aspect of metabolism is hydration. The metabolic processes can be greatly slowed down by dehydration since water is essential for nearly all chemical reactions in the body, including those that produce energy. Low energy, sluggish digestion, & less fat burning can all result from even moderate dehydration. In addition to sustaining metabolic processes, getting enough water throughout the day can help control hunger, which in turn can reduce the likelihood of overeating by reducing the intensity of needless cues for hunger. There is a role for the environment in metabolism as well. One example is how the body's energy expenditure is influenced by environmental temperature. Calorie expenditure can be enhanced in cold situations by non-shivering thermogenesis, which involves the body working harder to maintain its core temperature. Metabolic rate may also be affected by variations in the seasons. individuals have a tendency to put on more pounds as the weather becomes cold, but they might burn more calories when the weather gets warmer since more individuals are likely to be active. Sleep & stress are two of the most important aspects of health that influence metabolism. An imbalance in hormone control, impaired insulin sensitivity, & an increase in hunger hormones like ghrelin might cause weight gain if you don't get enough good sleep. A sluggish metabolism, an increased risk of obesity, & metabolic diseases are all linked to chronic sleep deprivation. Similarly, hormonal imbalances, especially increased cortisol levels, might promote fat accumulation & impede weight loss attempts when persistent stress is present. Keeping a healthy metabolism requires regular use of stress-reduction practices including meditation, yoga, & deep breathing. Lastly, metabolic function can be significantly affected by drugs & health problems. Medications for thyroid issues, antidepressants, & corticosteroids all interact with the body's energy systems in different ways, & some of these can have the opposite effect on metabolism. It can be challenging for individuals to maintain a healthy weight or energy levels when metabolic function is disrupted, as can happen with chronic illnesses such as diabetes, polycystic ovarian syndrome (PCOS), & metabolic syndrome. Restoration of metabolic equilibrium is possible through the medically supervised treatment of these underlying problems & the adoption of a holistic health strategy. Finally, many factors, both internal & external to the body, affect metabolism, making it a dynamic & intricate system. A person's metabolic rate is partly determined by their genes, but it can be improved or worsened by their lifestyle choices, including the amount of exercise they get, the food they eat, & the quality of sleep they get. In order to improve metabolism & maintain long-term health, individuals must understand how these elements interact, which is especially important when dealing with age, hormonal fluctuations, & underlying health issues, all of which further complicate metabolic processes. Maintaining a healthy metabolic rate & reducing the risk of metabolic dysfunction & related disorders can be achieved by a holistic approach that includes regular exercise, balanced eating, stress management, & appropriate sleep.

The Science of Energy Health

Energy health is the study of the complex processes that the body uses to turn food into energy, stay healthy, & keep balance by making sure that its metabolic & cellular systems work properly. The idea of metabolism is at the heart of energy health. Metabolism is the series of chemical reactions in the body that turn food into energy & build up the parts cells need to repair, grow, & work. Because they control how well the body makes & uses energy, these processes are not only necessary for survival but also for thriving. ATP, the body's energy currency, is made in the mitochondria, which are sometimes called the "powerhouses" of the cell. They take in nutrients like glucose & fatty acids & turn them into other molecules that the cell can use. Making ATP is an important part of energy health because it is needed for many things, like muscle contractions, nerve signals, & immune responses. The mitochondria are very complicated structures, & keeping them healthy is very important for making sure that the body keeps making energy. Genetics, diet, exercise, & environmental stressors are just some of the things that can help or hurt mitochondrial function. For example, foods that are high in antioxidants, healthy fats, & essential vitamins give mitochondria the building blocks they need to work. On the other hand, a sedentary lifestyle, bad nutrition, & environmental toxins can damage mitochondria, which can cause fatigue, a slowed metabolism, & disease. Energy balance is another important part of energy health. It's the relationship between how much energy we take in (from food & drink) & how much energy we use (through thermogenesis, physical activity, & basal metabolic rate). Getting & staying in balance with your energy is important for controlling your weight, improving your overall health, &

avoiding metabolic diseases. When you consistently take in more energy than you use, your body stores the extra calories as fat, which makes you gain weight. On the other hand, a chronic energy deficit can make you lose weight & muscle. To keep your energy levels & metabolism working at their best, you need to keep a balance between these two extremes. Hormones like insulin, leptin, & ghrelin, which control hunger, satiety, & fat storage, also have a big effect on how the body runs on energy.

Cellular Metabolism: How Energy is Created & Used

Cellular metabolism is the biochemical process by which nutrients are turned into energy. This energy is then used by cells to do many things, such as contracting muscles, making DNA, & keeping the body's balance. It works in every living cell & is very complicated & always changing. It is essential to life. The production & use of adenosine triphosphate (ATP), the cell's main source of energy, are at the heart of cellular metabolism. A group of metabolic pathways turn the chemical energy stored in nutrients, mostly glucose, fatty acids, & amino acids, into energy that the cell can use. Glycolysis starts the process. It happens in the cytoplasm of the cell & turns glucose into pyruvate & a small amount of ATP. Even though glycolysis is an anaerobic process (it doesn't need oxygen), the pyruvate it makes goes into the mitochondria to be used for more energy production. The second part of cellular metabolism takes place here: aerobic respiration. This process needs oxygen & happens in the mitochondria, which are the cell's "powerhouses." In the mitochondria, pyruvate changes in a process called the citric acid cycle, also called the Krebs cycle. During this process, pyruvate is changed into acetyl-CoA. This goes into the citric acid cycle & starts a chain of chemical reactions that free up high-energy electrons. The electron transport chain is made up of a group of protein complexes that are buried in the inner mitochondrial membrane. These electrons are moved through the chain, & their energy is used to make a lot of ATP. Either way, the electron transport chain makes water & a proton gradient, which powers ATP synthesis through a process called oxidative phosphorylation. Most of the ATP that cells need is made by this set of reactions, which includes the citric acid cycle & oxidative phosphorylation. But this very efficient process needs oxygen, which is why cells get their energy from aerobic respiration in places with lots of oxygen. Cells can switch to anaerobic metabolism if they don't have enough oxygen, but it works much less well. When cells don't have enough oxygen, like when they're working out hard or when they have a disease, they use glycolysis to make ATP. However, this process makes lactic acid, which can build up & make muscles tired. The role of fatty acid oxidation is another important part of cellular metabolism. Most of the time, glucose is the body's main source of energy, especially during times of high-intensity activity. However, fatty acids are the body's preferred energy source during times of rest or low-intensity activity. Triglycerides are a type of fat that the body stores fatty acids in. These can be broken down into free fatty acids & glycerol. Then, these free fatty acids go to the mitochondria, where they are broken down into two-carbon units through a process called beta-oxidation. Then, these units are changed into acetyl-CoA, which goes into the citric acid cycle & gives cells a lot of ATP. Metabolic flexibility is the ability of cells to quickly switch between burning glucose & fat. It is an important part of a healthy cell metabolism. Keeping this flexibility lets the body adjust to different energy needs &

situations, like when you're fasting, working out, or recovering. Along with the aerobic & anaerobic pathways for making ATP, amino acids from proteins also play a role in cellular metabolism. This happens less often, though, & usually only when glucose & fat stores are low. During digestion, proteins are first broken down into their individual amino acids. These amino acids can then be changed into different intermediates that can be used in the citric acid cycle to make ATP. When amino acids are turned into glucose, this process is called gluconeogenesis. When they are turned into ketone bodies, which can be used as an alternative energy source, like when you're fasting or working out for a long time, it's called ketogenesis. Cellular metabolism is tightly controlled by enzymes & hormones that check for cellular stress, energy needs, & the availability of nutrients. Key enzymes like hexokinase, pyruvate kinase, & ATP synthase control how metabolites move through different pathways. This makes sure that the production of ATP matches the energy needs of the cell. In the same way, hormones like insulin & glucagon, which are released by the pancreas, control how nutrients are used. When you eat, your body releases insulin, which helps store glucose in the form of glycogen in your liver & muscles. When you don't eat for a while, your body releases glucagon, which encourages the release of glucose from glycogen stores & the production of glucose from non-carbohydrate sources like amino acids. Keeping the balance between these two hormones is important for keeping blood sugar levels steady & making sure the body always has energy, even when food isn't nearby. Along with these macronutrients, micronutrients play an even more important role in the metabolism of cells. Minerals & vitamins are needed by many enzymes that work in metabolic pathways. For instance, B vitamins like niacin (vitamin B3), riboflavin (vitamin B2), & thiamine (vitamin

B1) are very important for making energy because they help turn fats, carbohydrates, & proteins into forms that the body can use. Magnesium, zinc, & iron are also very important for the electron transport chain & the function of mitochondria. They help enzymes that make ATP work properly. Lack of any of these micronutrients can make cellular metabolism less efficient, which can cause tiredness, problems making energy, & metabolic disorders. Temperature, the amount of oxygen available, & toxins are some of the outside factors that can change cellular metabolism. One example is hypoxia, a condition in which the body or a part of the body does not get enough oxygen. This can make cells rely more on anaerobic metabolism, which makes less ATP & builds up lactic acid. In the same way, being exposed to drugs, environmental toxins, or pollutants can damage mitochondria & mess up the flow of energy production, which can damage & break down cells. Exposure to these kinds of stressors over a long period of time can make metabolic diseases like obesity, type 2 diabetes, & heart disease more likely. Cells use energy for more than just basic metabolic tasks like breathing & keeping the body at the right temperature. They also use energy for more complex tasks like muscle contraction, nerve signaling, immune response, & tissue repair. When cells are under stress, like when they are hurt or inflamed, they need more energy to fix the damage & fight off pathogens. It's similar to how muscle cells make more ATP when they are working hard to support contraction & movement. Cellular metabolism is very well tuned to give the body just the right amount of energy at the right time. This lets the body adapt to changing needs without affecting its most important functions. In conclusion, cellular metabolism is a very complicated & effective process that lets the body make & use energy for many purposes. Every cell in the body depends on cellular metabolism to stay alive. It breaks down glucose & fatty acids & makes ATP in the mitochondria. A key part of overall health is the body's ability to change its metabolism based on different energy sources & conditions. If this process is hampered, it can cause fatigue, metabolic disorders, & even disease. A balanced diet, regular physical activity, stress management, & enough sleep are all important for keeping cellular metabolism at its best. These things also help the body make & use energy efficiently. Understanding how cellular metabolism works is important for maintaining good energy & avoiding illness because it gives people the power to make choices that improve metabolic function & boost vitality.

Mitochondria: The Powerhouses of Our Cells

In fact, mitochondria are so important to our cells that they are often called their "powerhouses." They make most of the energy our bodies need to stay alive. These very small but very complicated structures are very important to cellular metabolism because they turn nutrients from food into ATP, which is the cell's main source of energy. The mitochondria are different from the nucleus because they have their own DNA that is not the same as the DNA in the nucleus. They also copy themselves without following the cell's division cycle. Because of this, scientists think that mitochondria are evolutionary leftovers from bacteria that were eaten by ancestral eukaryotic cells in a relationship that was good for both sides. This endosymbiotic theory says that mitochondria were once independent living things that changed over time to become part of the cell, giving energy in exchange for a stable environment inside the host. In the mitochondria, the process of making energy starts with breaking down carbohydrates, fats, & proteins into smaller molecules like glucose & fatty acids. These molecules go into the mitochondria & go through a series of metabolic processes. The Krebs cycle, which is another name for the citric acid cycle, is the most important of these processes. This cycle turns acetyl-CoA, which comes from glucose or fatty acids, into high-energy electrons that are carried by electron carriers like NADH & FADH2. The electrons then move through the electron transport chain, which is made up of a group of protein complexes that are buried in the inner mitochondrial membrane. Their energy is used to move protons, which are hydrogen ions, across the membrane, which creates an electrochemical gradient. Potential energy is made by this gradient, which is like water behind a dam. ATP synthase, an enzyme that makes ATP, uses this potential energy. The last step in this process is the reduction of oxygen molecules to water. This is why mitochondria need oxygen so much, & aerobic respiration is their main way of making energy. Maintaining the body's energy balance depends on how well mitochondria work, & when they aren't working properly, the effects can be very bad. Many illnesses, like Alzheimer's & Parkinson's, are linked to problems with the mitochondria. These include heart diseases, diabetes, neurodegenerative diseases, & even getting older. One common sign of mitochondrial dysfunction is a decreased ability to make ATP. This causes energy deficits that show up as tiredness, weak muscles, & mental decline. In addition to making energy, mitochondria also play a key role in many other important cellular processes. They are very important for controlling apoptosis, which is the programmed death of cells. They do this by releasing proteins that set off a chain of events that kill the cell. This process is very important for keeping tissue homeostasis & getting rid of cells that are damaged or don't work right. Calcium signaling, which is important for controlling many cellular activities like muscle contraction, neurotransmitter release, & hormone secretion, is also helped by mitochondria. Furthermore, mitochondria play a part in making some hormones & controlling the metabolism of cells. Even though they are small, mitochondria are very active parts of cells that are always changing their shape, size, & location inside the cell in response to energy needs & changes in the environment. The process by which they can join together, split up, or form networks depends on what the cell needs. This is called mitochondrial fusion & fission. These processes give the mitochondria a way to stay healthy & adapt to changes in the amount of energy they need. When cells are stressed or damaged, mitochondria can also help keep the quality of the cells. More energy needs can speed up the process of mitochondrial biogenesis, which makes new mitochondria. Damaged mitochondria can be destroyed selectively through a process called mitophagy, which makes sure that only healthy, working mitochondria stay inside the cell. The mitochondria stay healthy & work properly for a long time thanks to this constant cycle of repair, renewal, & degradation. The number of mitochondria in a cell changes a lot depending on how much energy the cell needs. For instance, muscle cells have thousands of mitochondria because they need a lot of energy to contract. Skin cells, on the other hand, have fewer mitochondria because they don't need as much energy. Organs that are always working & need a steady supply of energy, like the heart, brain, & liver, have a lot of mitochondria. On the other hand, cells that don't need as much energy, like some types of blood cells, have fewer mitochondria. Many things, like genetics, diet, exercise, & toxins in the environment, can affect the health of our mitochondria. Mitochondrial diseases are caused by changes in the DNA of mitochondria. These diseases usually affect tissues & organs that need a lot of energy, like muscles & the nervous system. These changes can make it harder for mitochondria to make ATP, which can cause diseases like Leber's hereditary optic neuropathy or mitochondrial myopathy. Many mitochondrial diseases are passed down through families, but the way you live your life can also have a big effect on your mitochondrial health. A diet full of antioxidants, vitamins, & minerals gives mitochondria the building blocks they need to work at their best. Coenzyme Q10, B vitamins, magnesium, & omega-3 fatty acids are some of the nutrients that help the mitochondria make energy & protect against oxidative damage. But bad eating habits, like eating too many processed foods, sugars, & trans fats, can make mitochondrial dysfunction worse by making oxidative stress & inflammation worse. It has been shown that physical activity, especially aerobic exercise, can improve mitochondrial function by speeding up the production of new mitochondria & making energy production more efficient. Getting regular exercise can also boost the number of mitochondria in cells, which makes them stronger & gives them more energy. On the other hand, not moving around much can cause mitochondrial decline, which can make conditions like obesity, type 2 diabetes, & metabolic syndrome worse. Pollutants, pesticides, & heavy metals in the environment can also hurt mitochondria by increasing oxidative stress & making it harder for them to make ATP. Because they make energy, mitochondria are very vulnerable to oxidative damage. This is because energy production makes free radicals. Oxidative stress happens when free radicals build up faster than the cell can get rid of them. This damages cells & makes mitochondrial function worse. One thing that speeds up aging is that mitochondria become less efficient over time. This means that less energy is made & more damage is done by free radicals. One interesting area of study is mitochondrial therapy, which aims to improve mitochondrial function & fix problems with mitochondrial dysfunction. This can include changes to your lifestyle, like eating better, working out, & getting enough sleep, as well as new treatments that focus on protecting mitochondrial DNA, speeding up mitochondrial biogenesis, or making it easier for damaged mitochondria to be thrown out. Several studies have shown that compounds like nicotinamide riboside, resveratrol, & metformin can help keep mitochondria healthy. Researchers are now looking into how to use these compounds. Besides this, scientists are also looking into gene therapy & mitochondrial transplantation as ways to treat mitochondrial diseases & help old or sick cells make more energy. Despite the difficulties of studying & manipulating mitochondria, improving their function holds great promise for improving energy health, preventing diseases that come with getting older, & making people healthier overall. In conclusion, mitochondria are very important parts of cells because they make ATP, which gives cells most of the energy they need. Their job is very important for keeping cells healthy, keeping the metabolism in check, & meeting the energy needs of different organs & tissues. A lot of different diseases are connected to mitochondrial dysfunction, such as metabolic conditions, cardiovascular disease, & diseases that damage nerve cells. We can increase energy production, lower the risk of disease, & improve our overall health by learning how mitochondria work & making changes to our lifestyles that support mitochondrial health. Researchers are still looking into ways to treat mitochondrial diseases, which gives people around the world hope for better health & longer lives.

Metabolic Flexibility & Its Importance

In fact, mitochondria are so important to our cells that they are often called their "powerhouses." They make most of the energy our bodies need to stay alive. These very small but very complicated structures are very important to cellular metabolism because they turn nutrients from food into ATP, which is the cell's main source of energy. The mitochondria are different from the nucleus because they have their own DNA that is not the same as the DNA in the nucleus. They also copy themselves without following the cell's division cycle. Because of this, scientists think that mitochondria are evolutionary leftovers from bacteria that were eaten by ancestral eukaryotic cells in a relationship that was good for both sides. This endosymbiotic theory says that mitochondria were once independent living things that changed over time to become part of the cell, giving energy in exchange for a stable environment inside the host. In the mitochondria, the process of making energy starts with breaking down carbohydrates, fats, & proteins into smaller molecules like glucose & fatty acids. These molecules go into the mitochondria & go through a series of metabolic processes. The Krebs cycle, which is another name for the citric acid cycle, is the most important of these processes. This cycle turns acetyl-CoA, which comes from glucose or fatty acids, into high-energy electrons that are carried by electron carriers like NADH & $FADH_2$. The electrons then move through the electron transport chain, which is made up of a group of protein complexes that are buried in the inner mitochondrial membrane. Their energy is used to move protons, which are hydrogen ions, across the membrane, which creates an electrochemical gradient. Potential energy is made by this gradient, which is like water behind a dam.

ATP synthase, an enzyme that makes ATP, uses this potential energy. The last step in this process is the reduction of oxygen molecules to water. This is why mitochondria need oxygen so much, & aerobic respiration is their main way of making energy. Maintaining the body's energy balance depends on how well mitochondria work, & when they aren't working properly, the effects can be very bad. Many illnesses, like Alzheimer's & Parkinson's, are linked to problems with the mitochondria. These include heart diseases, diabetes, neurodegenerative diseases, & even getting older. One common sign of mitochondrial dysfunction is a decreased ability to make ATP. This causes energy deficits that show up as tiredness, weak muscles, & mental decline. In addition to making energy, mitochondria also play a key role in many other important cellular processes. They are very important for controlling apoptosis, which is the programmed death of cells. They do this by releasing proteins that set off a chain of events that kill the cell. This process is very important for keeping tissue homeostasis & getting rid of cells that are damaged or don't work right. Calcium signaling, which is important for controlling many cellular activities like muscle contraction, neurotransmitter release, & hormone secretion, is also helped by mitochondria. Furthermore, mitochondria play a part in making some hormones & controlling the metabolism of cells. Even though they are small, mitochondria are very active parts of cells that are always changing their shape, size, & location inside the cell in response to energy needs & changes in the environment. The process by which they can join together, split up, or form networks depends on what the cell needs. This is called mitochondrial fusion & fission. These processes give the mitochondria a way to stay healthy & adapt to changes in the amount of energy they need. When cells are stressed or damaged, mitochondria can also help keep the quality of the cells. More energy needs can speed up the process of mitochondrial biogenesis, which makes new mitochondria. Damaged mitochondria can be destroyed selectively through a process called mitophagy, which makes sure that only healthy, working mitochondria stay inside the cell. The mitochondria stay healthy & work properly for a long time thanks to this constant cycle of repair, renewal, & degradation. The number of mitochondria in a cell changes a lot depending on how much energy the cell needs. For instance, muscle cells have thousands of mitochondria because they need a lot of energy to contract. Skin cells, on the other hand, have fewer mitochondria because they don't need as much energy. Organs that are always working & need a steady supply of energy, like the heart, brain, & liver, have a lot of mitochondria. On the other hand, cells that don't need as much energy, like some types of blood cells, have fewer mitochondria. Many things, like genetics, diet, exercise, & toxins in the environment, can affect the health of our mitochondria. Mitochondrial diseases are caused by changes in the DNA of mitochondria. These diseases usually affect tissues & organs that need a lot of energy, like muscles & the nervous system. These changes can make it harder for mitochondria to make ATP, which can cause diseases like Leber's hereditary optic neuropathy or mitochondrial myopathy. Many mitochondrial diseases are passed down through families, but the way you live your life can also have a big effect on your mitochondrial health. A diet full of antioxidants, vitamins, & minerals gives mitochondria the building blocks they need to work at their best. Coenzyme Q10, B vitamins, magnesium, & omega-3 fatty acids are some of the nutrients that help the mitochondria make energy & protect against oxidative damage. But bad eating habits, like eating too many processed foods, sugars, & trans fats, can make mitochondrial dysfunction worse by making oxidative stress & inflammation worse. It has been shown that physical activity, especially aerobic exercise, can improve mitochondrial function by speeding up the production of new mitochondria & making energy production more efficient. Getting regular exercise can also boost the number of mitochondria in cells, which makes them stronger & gives them more energy. On the other hand, not moving around much can cause mitochondrial decline, which can make conditions like obesity, type 2 diabetes, & metabolic syndrome worse. Pollutants, pesticides, & heavy metals in the environment can also hurt mitochondria by increasing oxidative stress & making it harder for them to make ATP. Because they make energy, mitochondria are very vulnerable to oxidative damage. This is because energy production makes free radicals. Oxidative stress happens when free radicals build up faster than the cell can get rid of them. This damages cells & makes mitochondrial function worse. One thing that speeds up aging is that mitochondria become less efficient over time. This means that less energy is made & more damage is done by free radicals. One interesting area of study is mitochondrial therapy, which aims to improve mitochondrial function & fix problems with mitochondrial dysfunction. This can include changes to your lifestyle, like eating better, working out, & getting enough sleep, as well as new treatments that focus on protecting mitochondrial DNA, speeding up mitochondrial biogenesis, or making it easier for damaged mitochondria to be thrown out. Several studies have shown that compounds like nicotinamide riboside, resveratrol, & metformin can help keep mitochondria healthy. Researchers are now looking into how to use these compounds. Besides this, scientists are also looking into gene therapy & mitochondrial transplantation as ways to treat mitochondrial diseases & help old or sick cells make more energy. Despite the difficulties of studying & manipulating mitochondria, improving their function holds great promise for improving energy health, preventing diseases that come with getting older, & making people healthier overall. In conclusion, mitochondria are very important parts of cells because they make ATP, which gives cells most of the energy they need. Their job is very important for keeping cells healthy, keeping the metabolism in check, & meeting the energy needs of different organs & tissues. A lot of different diseases are connected to mitochondrial dysfunction, such as metabolic conditions, cardiovascular disease, & diseases that damage nerve cells. We can increase energy production, lower the risk of disease, & improve our overall health by learning how mitochondria work & making changes to our lifestyles that support mitochondrial health. Researchers are still looking into ways to treat mitochondrial diseases, which gives people around the world hope for better health & longer lives.

Metabolism & Your Immune System

The metabolic process affects the immune system's function, & the immune system's responses shape metabolic activity. The immune system protects the body from harmful invaders, while metabolism essentially consists of chemical reactions that transform food into energy, control energy expenditure, & keep the body at a constant internal temperature (homeostasis). You see, these two systems aren't independent of each other; in fact, they're vital to your health because of the dynamic & mutually beneficial relationship they share. The production & control of energy is one of the principal mechanisms by which metabolism affects immune function. Just like any other kind of cell in the body, immune cells need energy to carry out their duties. A steady flow of energy is essential for the functioning of all immune cells, including white blood cells (such as T cells, B cells, macrophages, & neutrophils) that scour the body for invaders & dendritic cells & macrophages that react to infections. The metabolic processes that supply energy to immune cells are affected by factors such as the body's nutritional status, hormonal signals, & the availability of nutrients. The immune system changes its metabolism to accommodate the increased metabolic demands that occur during an immune response. To counteract infections or injuries, for instance, immune cells speed up their metabolic rate to fuel the inflammatory response, encourage the production of signaling molecules like cytokines, & facilitate quick proliferation & differentiation to fend off the invader. This is demonstrated by the fact that macrophages & T lymphocytes undergo substantial metabolic changes when they become activated during an infection. Critical to immune cell function are metabolic changes that take place during activation; for example, immune cells may move away from oxidative phosphorylation, the main energy-producing process for most cells under normal circumstances, & toward glycolysis, which generates ATP rapidly in the absence of oxygen, enabling immune cells to react swiftly to threats. Inflammation & infection cause immune cells to undergo metabolic reprogramming, which includes this switch. The tight relationship between metabolism & immune function is further demonstrated by this metabolic change, which aids immune cells in meeting their increased energy demands. Conversely, metabolic processes are also susceptible to immune system influence. One example is the secretion of cytokines, which are signaling molecules that regulate the activity of immune cells & other tissues, when the immune system is activated in response to an infection or inflammation. Tumor necrosis factor-alpha (TNF-α) is a famous cytokine that has been linked to metabolic alterations in inflammatory conditions. The metabolic activity of adipose tissue (fat cells), liver, & muscle cells can be impacted by TNF-α & other pro-inflammatory cytokines, resulting in changes to lipid metabolism, insulin resistance, & altered glucose metabolism. Metabolic dysregulation can persist in conditions characterized by chronic inflammation, such as autoimmune disorders, obesity, & type 2 diabetes. An example of this is the vicious cycle of metabolic dysfunction that develops when adipose tissue becomes inflamed in obesity. This inflammation leads to higher levels of pro-inflammatory cytokines, which in turn impair insulin sensitivity & glucose metabolism. An individual's nutritional status is an important factor in determining the efficacy of immune responses, in addition to the direct effects of immune activation on metabolism. The immune system cannot work properly without certain nutrients. These include carbs, proteins, fats, vitamins, & minerals. For example, the activation of immune cells requires vitamin D, zinc, & iron, while the proliferation & function of immune cells depend on amino acids such as arginine & glutamine. Impairments in immune responses caused by nutrient deficiencies can make people more susceptible to infections & take longer to recover from them. Conversely, metabolic diseases can develop when specific nutrients, particularly sugars & lipids, are consumed in excess, leading to chronic low-grade inflammation that suppresses the immune system. So, to keep oneself healthy all the time, one must eat a well-balanced diet that helps the immune system & metabolism. In the setting of an infection, the involvement of metabolism in immune responses becomes even more apparent. In the midst of an infection, the immune system goes into overdrive, setting off an inflammatory response that involves a myriad of metabolic changes & targets the invading pathogen specifically. The acute phase response is one example of a metabolic change that occurs in response to infection or injury. It entails changes in glucose & lipid metabolism as well as an increase in the production of specific proteins by the liver, such as C-reactive protein (CRP). The immune response & this metabolic change work together to refocus energy on warding off the infection & mending injured tissues. It is believed that the immune system-driven metabolic changes cause fever, a common symptom of infection, by making the body's environment less favorable for pathogen survival. A proper immune response requires metabolic reprogramming, which can be taxing on the body. In the case of long-term illnesses, the interplay between the immune system & metabolism becomes even more important. Heart disease, cancer, & neurological disorders are just a few of the many diseases & conditions that have been associated to chronic inflammation, which is frequently caused by metabolic dysfunction. The development of insulin resistance—a state in which cells in the body become less responsive to insulin, resulting in elevated blood glucose levels—contributes to metabolic diseases like type 2 diabetes, for example, chronic low-grade inflammation. People with metabolic diseases are more likely to get infections because inflammation lowers immune function. Alternatively, metabolic health can be improved through weight management, exercise, & dietary changes, which can aid in reducing chronic inflammation, restoring immune function, & lowering disease risk. Metabolic & immunological function are two areas where exercise is very important regulators. Exercising on a regular basis lowers markers of chronic inflammation, increases insulin sensitivity, & improves metabolic flexibility. In addition to boosting the body's capacity to fend off infections, exercise boosts the immune system by increasing the flow of immune cells throughout the body & making immune cells like T cells & macrophages work better. Some research suggests that the metabolic changes brought about by exercise, like better mitochondrial function & increased fat oxidation, help the immune system by supplying the energy that immune cells need to do their jobs. Additionally, there is a strong correlation between immune function & gut health, & exercise has been demonstrated to enhance both. The trillions of bacteria that call the digestive tract home make up the gut microbiome, & they're vital for metabolic control & immune system homeostasis. Digestive health, nutrient absorption, & immunological function are all enhanced by a balanced gut microbiome. The significance of gut health in relation to metabolism & immunity is highlighted by the fact that dysbiosis, defined as an imbalance in the gut microbiome, has been linked to metabolic disorders as well as immune dysfunction. New studies have also shown that autophagy, the body's mechanism for removing damaged cells & making replacements, may play a role in bridging the gap between metabolism & immunity. Crucial for immune function & metabolic regulation, autophagy aids in cellular health maintenance by removing dysfunctional proteins & mitochondria. Metabolic disorders & immune system dysfunction have been associated with impaired autophagy; therefore, increasing autophagic activity by means of lifestyle interventions like exercise & fasting may enhance metabolic & immune health. Finally, both the immune system & metabolism are highly dependent on one another for proper functioning & control. The metabolic processes play a crucial role in meeting the energy needs of immune cells, & when the immune system is activated, especially during inflammation, it can greatly affect these processes. A vicious cycle of chronic inflammation & metabolic dysfunction can worsen immune system imbalances & metabolic abnormalities, leaving the body more vulnerable to illness. Key tactics for supporting metabolic & immune health include eating a balanced diet, exercising regularly, & managing stress. While regulating metabolism & lowering the risk of metabolic diseases are both aided by immune system optimization, individuals can improve their immune system's response to infections & illnesses by optimizing metabolic function. Because of the interconnected nature of metabolism & immunity, it is crucial to take a holistic view of health that takes into account both systems. This will help build a body that is better able to avoid & overcome diseases.

How a Healthy Metabolism Protects Against Disease

The regulation of the body's energy balance, the promotion of cellular function, & the protection against various chronic diseases are all functions of a healthy metabolism, which is essential for optimal health. Metabolic pathways are the intricate web of intracellular chemical reactions that facilitate energy production, tissue repair, & the myriad other vital physiological functions. Many aspects of health are dependent on the metabolic system's efficiency & flexibility, including the regulation of body weight, the functioning of the immune system, & the capacity to recover from injuries & infections. The ability to adapt to fluctuating energy needs, efficiently store & use nutrients, & sustain homeostasis (a condition of stable internal conditions) all depend on a metabolic system that is working properly. By maintaining normal insulin sensitivity & controlling blood sugar levels, a healthy metabolism largely shields the body from disease. The pancreas secretes the hormone insulin, which aids in glucose regulation by allowing cells to take glucose in for energy production or storage. Conditions like type 2 diabetes, in which the body develops a resistance to insulin, cause blood glucose levels to stay high, which in turn increases the risk of cardiovascular disease, kidney damage, nerve damage, & other consequences. However, insulin sensitivity is preserved in a metabolically sound body, which permits steady blood sugar levels & efficient glucose uptake. This lowers the risk of developing diabetes & a host of other complications associated with long-term high blood sugar levels. In addition, the cardiovascular system's proper operation is intimately related to metabolic health. Proper regulation of lipid metabolism is essential for maintaining a healthy blood fat balance, & a healthy metabolism helps to achieve this goal. While lipids like cholesterol & triglycerides are necessary for cells to work, metabolic dysfunction (which can result from things like an unhealthy diet, not getting enough exercise, & being overweight) causes the body to make too much "bad" cholesterol, or low-density lipoprotein (LDL) cholesterol, which can cause plaque to build up in the arteries & raise the risk of atherosclerosis (the hardening of the arteries), heart attacks, & strokes. Keeping cholesterol levels in check & protecting against cardiovascular diseases are both aided by a healthy metabolism's emphasis on lipid metabolism. Weight management is an important component in illness prevention, & a healthy metabolism aids in this endeavor. Numerous chronic diseases, such as type 2 diabetes, heart disease, & some cancers, are greatly increased in prevalence when people are overweight, which is frequently caused by an imbalance in the metabolic system. When the metabolic system is working properly, fat is used & stored appropriately; this keeps the body from storing too much fat, especially visceral fat, which is located around important organs like the pancreas & liver. Metabolic syndrome is a group of symptoms that includes hypertension, diabetes, high cholesterol, & excess abdominal fat. When visceral fat is excessive, it triggers the release of inflammatory chemicals & hormones that hinder insulin function, encourage additional fat storage, & raise the risk of these complications. Keeping to a healthy weight & achieving an ideal distribution of fat can help keep these risks at bay & lower the chances of developing metabolic diseases. Maintaining immune function & reducing inflammation are two important components in disease prevention, & a healthy metabolism is essential for all three. It also controls blood sugar & fat metabolism. Metabolic health is associated with optimal energy production & utilization by the immune system, which in turn protects the body from infections, viruses, & other dangerous pathogens. White blood cells, macrophages, & T lymphocytes—all components of the immune system—need a strong metabolism to properly identify & destroy foreign invaders. Metabolic syndrome & obesity, on the other hand, cause persistent low-grade inflammation that compromises immunity & raises the risk of cancer, autoimmune illnesses, & infections. Although inflammation is an immune system reaction to pathogens or injuries, it can lead to various diseases when it persists over an extended period of time & damages vital organs & tissues. By maintaining a steady equilibrium between pro- & anti-inflammatory molecules, a metabolically sound body can control inflammatory responses, limiting the occurrence of chronic inflammation & making sure the immune system responds only when called upon. Repair & regeneration of cells rely heavily on metabolism, which is involved in immune function as well. Metabolic energy is essential for the continual cellular repair, regeneration, & replacement that occurs in the body. At its best, the metabolic process facilitates the synthesis of adenosine triphosphate (ATP), the universal energy currency required for all cellular processes, including DNA replication, cellular repair, & tissue regeneration. In addition, most of the ATP utilized in cellular processes is produced by the mitochondria, which are commonly called the cell's powerhouses. Efficient energy production by mitochondria is a hallmark of a healthy metabolism, which in turn helps cells maintain & repair themselves, warding off cellular damage that can hasten aging, cancer, & degenerative diseases. Metabolic health is paramount when considering the aging process. A slower metabolic rate is associated with age-related changes in lean body mass, fat distribution, & energy homeostasis. Deterioration of mitochondrial function, which hinders cellular maintenance & energy generation, is another hallmark of aging. By enhancing mitochondrial function, preserving muscle mass, & supporting overall cellular health, a healthy metabolism—supported by regular physical activity, a balanced diet, & proper sleep—can help to slow down the aging process. One way to ward off age-related ailments like osteoporosis, sarcopenia (muscle atrophy), & neurodegenerative diseases like Alzheimer's is to keep one's metabolism in good shape all through life. Metabolic regulation of hormones is another important part of metabolism's function in illness prevention. Growth, mood, metabolism, & reproductive health are just a few of the many bodily functions influenced by hormones, which are chemical messengers. Key hormones in regulating metabolism include insulin, thyroid, cortisol, & sex hormones. As an example, thyroid hormones control the rate of energy production from food by regulating the speed of metabolism. Weight gain, lethargy, cardiovascular issues, & mental health issues are just some of the symptoms that can arise from a thyroid gland that is either underactive (hypothyroidism) or overactive (hyperthyroidism). The stress hormone cortisol is also essential for metabolic regulation, especially under stressful conditions. Sustained high levels of cortisol, which can be caused by chronic stress, can impair immune function, increase abdominal fat storage, & disrupt metabolic processes. Ensuring that hormone levels remain within healthy ranges through maintaining a balanced metabolism helps to prevent disorders & diseases related to hormones. Optimal brain function & mental health are also dependent on a healthy metabolism. As a high-energy organ, the brain relies heavily on the efficient metabolism of lipids & glucose to carry out its functions. Impaired metabolism, such as insulin resistance, hinders the brain's capacity to absorb glucose & other nutrients, resulting in cognitive impairment, impaired memory, & an elevated risk of neurodegenerative disorders such as Alzheimer's & Parkinson's. A healthy metabolism protects against mental health disorders & cognitive decline by supporting the brain's metabolic needs. A healthy metabolism not only aids in the prevention of chronic diseases, but it also promotes general vitality & wellness. Having a well-regulated metabolic system is associated with many health benefits, including more energy, improved mood, better sleep, & greater physical performance. A more efficient use of energy by the body leads to improved fitness, quicker recovery from exercise, & longer durations of physical activity. A healthy lifestyle is crucial for preventing diseases, & this encourages just that. Keeping up a regular exercise routine, eating well, managing stress, & getting enough sleep all help keep metabolic health in check & lower the risk of disease. Finally, a healthy metabolism safeguards the body from numerous chronic diseases, such as type 2 diabetes, heart disease, obesity, cancer, & neurological disorders. Maintaining homeostasis & preventing disease are roles played by a properly functioning metabolism, which efficiently manages energy production, regulates blood sugar & lipid levels, supports immune function, reduces inflammation, & promotes cellular repair. Optimal metabolic health is the result of a combination of factors that contribute to general wellness, such as a healthy diet, regular exercise, enough sleep, & stress management. People can live longer, better lives, & experience fewer health problems if they put metabolic health first.

The Connection Between Metabolism & Inflammation

An important part of learning how the body deals with stress, infections, & chronic diseases is delving into the link between inflammation & metabolism. The metabolic pathway is the network of chemical reactions that the body uses to generate energy from food, sustain cellular function, & keep itself healthy. But inflammation is the immune system's way of dealing with harmful stimuli, infections, or injuries. Although short-lived inflammation plays an important role in the immune system's defense mechanism, long-term inflammation is a disease that can cause numerous health issues. Crucially, there is a complicated & ever-changing relationship between inflammation & metabolism. The two are strongly related. The body's inflammatory responses can be better managed with a healthy metabolism, but metabolic diseases & their complications can develop when inflammation has a negative impact on metabolic function.

The idea of the energy requirements of immune cells is fundamental to the relationship between inflammation & metabolism. The body's immune system is able to detect & respond to infections & injuries by activating & mobilizing cells like macrophages, neutrophils, & T-cells. Energy is essential for these immune cells to perform their tasks, such as producing cytokines that control the inflammatory response. Metabolic reactions such as glycolysis, oxidative phosphorylation, & fatty acid oxidation source this energy. There is a metabolic switch occurring in immune cells during acute inflammation from the oxygen-dependent & more efficient oxidative phosphorylation to the faster & less efficient anaerobic glycolysis. Inflammatory responses like cytokine release, phagocytosis, & cell proliferation rely on immune cells rapidly producing ATP, which is made possible by this change. The body's immune cells are able to fight infections, restore damaged tissues, & safeguard the body from harmful pathogens because of metabolic reprogramming.

On the other hand, metabolic dysfunction is a common cause of chronic inflammation, which in turn can have major impacts on metabolic processes, leading to a self-perpetuating cycle that worsens metabolic dysfunction & inflammation. Metabolic disorders, including obesity, type 2 diabetes, & cardiovascular disease, are characterized by chronic low-grade inflammation. Adipose tissue (fat) inflammation & increased release of pro-inflammatory cytokines characterize these diseases. Normal metabolic processes are disrupted by cytokines like tumor necrosis factor-alpha (TNF-α) & interleukin-6 (IL-6). As an illustration, research has demonstrated that TNF-α hinders insulin signaling by increasing insulin resistance in various tissues such as muscle, liver, & adipose tissue. This, in turn, causes problems with glucose metabolism & ultimately leads to elevated blood sugar levels. Metabolic diseases like type 2 diabetes can develop as a result of this. In addition to damaging cells, tissues, & organs via oxidative stress, pro-inflammatory cytokines can boost ROS production.

Visceral fat, a type of adipose tissue that surrounds important organs, plays a significant role in the relationship between inflammation & metabolism. Visceral fat, in contrast to the more inert subcutaneous fat just under the skin, is metabolically active & capable of secreting a wide range of chemicals, such as adipokines & cytokines. Adipose tissue aids a healthy metabolism by storing energy as fat & releasing it when needed. Nevertheless, inflammatory cytokines like TNF-α, IL-6, & C-reactive protein (CRP) are produced in individuals with metabolic syndrome or obesity due to an excess of visceral fat. Insulin resistance & additional metabolic dysfunction are outcomes of these cytokines' interference with insulin sensitivity, which in turn promotes systemic inflammation. Conditions such as diabetes, high blood pressure, & heart disease can develop as a result of this process.

Inflammation impacts other metabolically active tissues besides adipose tissue, including the pancreas, muscles, & liver. Fat buildup & the onset of non-alcoholic fatty liver disease (NAFLD) can result from impaired lipid metabolism in the liver caused by chronic inflammation. Inflammation in muscles can reduce calorie burning by blocking the oxidation of glucose & fat. Damage to insulin-producing beta cells in the pancreas due to inflammation can make insulin resistance even worse & raise the risk of developing type 2 diabetes.

How much inflammation becomes chronic is influenced by metabolic health, which is an interesting finding. One powerful anti-inflammatory agent is regular physical activity. Exercising improves metabolic flexibility, which means the body can use fats & carbohydrates for energy depending on what's available. This metabolic flexibility aids in inflammation regulation by decreasing fat storage & increasing the secretion of adiponectin, which are anti-inflammatory chemicals. Supporting a healthy equilibrium between inflammation & metabolism, exercise has additional benefits, such as improving immune cell function & reducing the production of pro-inflammatory cytokines.

When it comes to the link between metabolism & inflammation, nutrition is also very important. Inflammation can be worsened by eating a lot of processed foods, refined sugars, & bad fats, but it can be alleviated by eating lots of fresh produce, whole grains, & healthy fats (such as nuts, olive oil, & fatty fish). Metabolic health is supported by nutrients that have anti-inflammatory properties, such as polyphenols, antioxidants, & omega-3 fatty acids. On the flip side, metabolic diseases can develop in people whose diets are heavy in refined carbs & saturated fats, which raise levels of cytokines that promote inflammation.

In addition to food & exercise, other aspects of one's lifestyle, like stress & sleep, can impact the connection between inflammation & metabolism. The production of the hormone cortisol, which can enhance inflammation & promote fat storage, is triggered by the body's fight-or-flight response when chronic stress is present. Insulin resistance, visceral fat accumulation, & metabolic disease risk factors are all exacerbated by prolonged exposure to high cortisol levels. Conversely, regulating inflammatory processes & keeping metabolic health in check depend on getting enough sleep. Research has demonstrated that insufficient or poor quality sleep can worsen inflammation & metabolic dysfunction by increasing the production of cytokines that promote inflammation & by hindering glucose metabolism.

To maintain a healthy equilibrium between energy production & immune responses, signaling pathways control inflammation & metabolism at the cellular level. During inflammatory responses, the nuclear factor kappa B (NF-κB) pathway is activated, making it one of the important regulators of inflammation & metabolism. Insulin resistance, fat storage, & glucose metabolism are all regulated by NF-κB, which is also involved in the production of pro-inflammatory cytokines. Normal metabolic processes can be disturbed & chronic diseases can be worsened when inflammation activates NF-κB. Restoring metabolic balance & reducing the risk of metabolic diseases can be achieved through interventions that decrease NF-κB activation, such as anti-inflammatory medications, exercise, & a nutritious diet.

The gut microbiome, a complex network of microbes found in the digestive tract, is another important actor in the metabolism-inflammation connection. Through its effects on immune function, nutrient absorption, & the synthesis of molecules that modulate inflammation, the gut microbiome is an important metabolic & inflammatory regulator. Metabolic dysfunction & chronic inflammation have both been associated with dysbiosis, which is an imbalance in the gut microbiome. One example is "leaky gut," a condition where inflammatory molecules leak into the bloodstream due to an imbalance in gut bacteria that increases the permeability of the gut lining. Obesity, type 2 diabetes, & cardiovascular disease are worsened metabolic function & risk is increased when systemic inflammation is triggered.

In conclusion, there is a great deal of reciprocal influence between metabolism & inflammation. Assuring that immune cells have the energy to battle infections & repair tissue damage, a healthy metabolism also helps to regulate the body's inflammatory response, which in turn helps to prevent metabolic diseases caused by chronic low-grade inflammation. Metabolic dysfunction, which can be brought on by things like being overweight, eating poorly, not getting enough exercise, & dealing with chronic stress, can lead to chronic inflammation, which in turn can amplify metabolic & immune system imbalances. Individuals can play a role in breaking this cycle & reducing the risk of inflammation-related diseases by promoting metabolic health through food, exercise, stress management, & sleep. To develop strategies to prevent & treat chronic conditions & promote overall health & longevity, it is essential to understand the complex relationship between inflammation & metabolism.

Balancing Metabolism for Immune Health

The immune system relies on a well-regulated metabolism to support overall health. Metabolism controls energy production, immune cell function, & inflammatory responses. The body's metabolic processes, which include digestion, energy storage, & nutrient conversion, supply the fuel that immune cells need to carry out their duties effectively. Lymphocytes, macrophages, & dendritic cells are just a few examples of immune cells that rely on the energy generated by metabolic reactions to carry out their various roles. Because of their role in identifying & eliminating infectious microbes, these cells play an essential defensive role in the body. The proliferation, migration, & execution of immune responses such as phagocytosis (the engulfing & digestion of pathogens) & cytokine production—signaling molecules that modulate immune activity—require an adequate supply of energy, similar to the energy required for muscular contractions. Immune cells may not work as well if the metabolism isn't stable & efficient, which can make the body more susceptible to infections & slow down the healing process after injuries. The proper functioning of the immune system depends on a metabolically balanced system that coordinates the production of energy through pathways like glycolysis, oxidative phosphorylation, & fatty acid oxidation. For instance, when faced with an infection or injury, immune cells replace the oxygen-efficient aerobic respiration with the faster but less efficient glycolysis to produce energy. This change can only take place when the metabolism is under control, which is essential for quick immune responses & cell proliferation. Metabolic efficiency is also critical for the synthesis of ATP, the cell's principal energy currency, which provides immune cells with the fuel they need to fight infections & carry out their homeostatic duties. The immune system's responsiveness to stresses is compromised in metabolic disorders like metabolic syndrome, obesity, or diabetes, which makes the body less capable of defending itself against illnesses. Important molecules that control immune function, cytokines, can tilt one way or the other under these circumstances. Chronic low-grade inflammation results from this imbalance; this inflammation has an adaptive role in fighting infections, but it can become harmful & contribute to autoimmune disorders & chronic diseases when left unchecked. Rheumatoid arthritis, lupus, & other autoimmune diseases are caused by the immune system being unable to differentiate between harmful pathogens & the body's own tissues due to chronic inflammation. The opposite is true for an optimized metabolism, which guarantees efficient allocation of energy resources, promotes effective immune responses, & maintains a balance between inflammatory signals & chronic inflammation. Engaging in regular physical activity is a powerful strategy to promote a healthy metabolism & immune system. Increased metabolic flexibility, or the capacity to use both carbs & fats as fuel, is one of the many benefits of exercise. This includes better mitochondrial function, more efficient energy production, & immune system support. To combat chronic inflammation, exercise increases the production of adiponectin & other anti-inflammatory molecules & increases the capacity of mitochondria, the cellular powerhouses, to produce ATP. In addition, physical exercise boosts immunity by increasing cell production & improving cell circulation, which in turn improves the body's capacity to detect & combat infections. Because metabolic function & immune responses typically decrease with age, this becomes even more crucial when considering the aging process. By keeping your metabolism & immune system in check, regular exercise can halt this deterioration. To maintain a healthy metabolism & immune system, nutrition is an important ally. Fruits, vegetables, whole grains, lean meats, & healthy fats are all part of a balanced diet that helps keep cells healthy & the metabolism running smoothly by providing antioxidants, vitamins, & minerals. The immune system relies on certain nutrients for proper functioning. Zinc, vitamin D, & omega-3 fatty acids are some of these nutrients. They help regulate the body's inflammatory response & promote the development & maintenance of immune cells. Conversely, metabolic imbalance, inflammation, & impaired immune cell function can result from a diet heavy in processed foods, refined sugars, & unhealthy fats. Overconsumption of refined carbs & bad fats, particularly trans fats, lowers insulin sensitivity & boosts pro-inflammatory cytokine production, all of which weaken the immune system. People can support immune function & lower their risk of chronic diseases by promoting a healthy metabolism through nutrient balance & avoiding inflammatory foods. A healthy metabolism is essential for a strong immune system, & other lifestyle factors like getting enough sleep & managing stress are just as important. When you sleep, your body releases hormones that regulate your metabolism, which in turn affects your hunger, energy expenditure, & immune response. Insulin resistance, impaired glucose metabolism, & elevated levels of the stress hormone cortisol are metabolic disturbances brought about by insufficient or poor-quality sleep. The body becomes more prone to infections when cortisol levels are elevated, which is caused by chronic stress. People can help maintain metabolic balance & increase their immune system's resistance to infections by making restorative sleep a priority. In a similar vein, lowering the chronic elevation of cortisol through stress management practices like yoga, meditation, or mindfulness can aid in maintaining a balanced metabolic state. In addition to improving immune responses & decreasing inflammation, this has a multiplicative effect on health & illness prevention. A cell's metabolic health is intricately related to the homeostasis of critical molecules that control inflammation. A key molecule in this category is AMP-activated protein kinase (AMPK), which is involved in cellular energy sensing. In response to low energy conditions, AMPK helps cells respond by starting processes that restore energy balance, such as increasing glucose uptake & fatty acid oxidation. It acts as a metabolic regulator. One important regulator of the inflammatory response, AMPK can inhibit the activation of the NF-κB pathway, which means it also has anti-inflammatory effects. Encouraging energy efficiency & immune system regulation, AMPK activity is optimized by maintaining a balanced metabolism. The SIRT1 protein, which belongs to the sirtuin family of enzymes, has been demonstrated to promote immune function & metabolic health in a similar vein. By deacetylating critical transcription factors involved in immune responses, SIRT1 aids in inflammation regulation & promotes mitochondrial function, both of which are essential for energy production. Reducing inflammation & supporting immune health, activating SIRT1 through calorie restriction, exercise, & specific dietary components (such as resveratrol in red wine & grapes) can improve metabolism & immune function. The role of the gut microbiome in regulating inflammation & metabolism extends well beyond these molecular pathways. Because the gastrointestinal tract (gut) is where the immune system primarily operates, the trillions of bacteria that live there affect metabolic processes as well as immune responses. Dysbiosis, an imbalance of gut bacteria linked to chronic inflammation & metabolic dysfunction, can't occur unless the gut microbiome is diverse & well-balanced, which in turn regulates immune system function & promotes the production of anti-inflammatory molecules. An optimal gut microbiome aids in nutrient metabolism, the synthesis of immune cells, & the production of short-chain fatty acids, which reduce inflammation. On the flip side, "leaky gut" occurs when there is an imbalance of bacteria in the gut & the intestinal lining becomes more permeable. This opens the door for harmful bacteria & inflammatory molecules to enter the bloodstream, where they can cause systemic inflammation & metabolic dysfunction. In order to keep metabolism & immune system in check, it is essential to maintain a balanced gut microbiome through food, probiotics, & prebiotics. To sum up, maintaining a healthy immune system begins with a balanced metabolism. To effectively fight off infections, inflammation, & disease, the body relies on its immune cells, which in turn rely on a metabolic system that is well-regulated. But when metabolism goes awry, as it does in metabolic syndrome, obesity, or insulin resistance, the immune system gets dysregulated, which causes chronic inflammation & raises the risk of many diseases, such as autoimmune disorders, cancer, heart disease, & cardiovascular disease. People can take care of their metabolism, inflammation, & immune system by making healthy lifestyle choices like exercising regularly, eating a balanced diet, managing their stress, & getting enough sleep. To further improve the relationship between metabolism & immune health, which promotes long-term wellness & disease prevention, it is important to maintain a balanced gut microbiome & support key metabolic pathways. Finally, keeping the immune system strong & able to defend the body from infections & other health threats depends on a balanced metabolism, which is critical for energy regulation.

Key Factors that Influence Metabolism

There is a myriad of factors that impact metabolism, the series of biochemical reactions that take place in the body to transform food into energy & sustain life. Impacting the body's calorie-burning, hormone-regulating, & health-maintaining metabolic functions, these factors can either help or hurt metabolic function. Age, gender, heredity, lean body mass, exercise, nutrition, hormone regulation, rest, stress, & environmental variables are among the most influential aspects of metabolism. The body's ability to process nutrients, produce energy, & keep itself at a constant temperature depends critically on each of these factors. Among the most important variables influencing metabolism is age. Changes in body composition, including a loss of muscle mass & an increase in fat mass, cause metabolic rates to decrease with age. The metabolic rate of muscle tissue is higher than that of fat tissue, so an individual's resting metabolic rate increases in direct proportion to their muscle mass. Because their metabolism gets less efficient with age, many people in their twilight years gain weight or find it difficult to lose weight. Muscle atrophy & the natural decline in growth hormone & testosterone levels that comes with getting older are two of the main causes of a sluggish metabolic rate. Another important component of metabolic rate variations is gender. As a general rule, men's metabolic rates are higher than women's because of their bigger stature & more muscular mass. A higher resting metabolic rate is one of the many benefits of testosterone, the principal male sex hormone, which aids in the growth & preservation of muscular mass. On the other hand, women tend to have a lower metabolic rate due to their higher proportion of fat, which is not as metabolically active as muscle tissue. Metabolic function is also greatly influenced by heredity. There are a number of hereditary variables that control thermogenesis (the body's process of producing heat & burning calories), which can affect whether an individual has a fast or slow metabolism. There is a strong correlation between variations in genes that regulate mitochondrial function & the efficiency with which the body generates energy. In addition, the way the body reacts to changes in food, exercise, & environmental factors may be influenced by specific genetic variations. For instance, some people may find it more difficult to lose weight due to a genetic tendency to store fat more efficiently. Another important component that affects metabolism is muscle mass. Even when at rest, muscle tissue continues to burn more calories than fat tissue. The amount of calories required to sustain basic bodily functions while at rest is known as the basal metabolic rate (BMR), & it is generally higher in people who have a higher percentage of muscle mass. Building muscle through consistent resistance training & strength training speeds up the metabolic rate. Although aerobic activities such as jogging & cycling help maintain heart health & burn calories while exercising, the best approach to gain muscle & improve metabolic function over time is strength training. Exercise & regular movement both contribute significantly to a healthy metabolism. Excess post-exercise oxygen consumption (EPOC) is a metabolic byproduct of exercise that increases energy expenditure both during & after physical activity. The term for this phenomenon, which occurs when the body's calorie-burning rate remains elevated after a workout, aids in the acceleration of fat loss, is the "afterburn" effect. The extent to which EPOC affects metabolism is dependent on exercise intensity, duration, & type. Because it involves short bursts of intense exercise separated by rest or lower-intensity activity, high-intensity interval training (HIIT) is great at raising metabolic rate. Walking, standing, & fidgeting are examples of everyday physical activity that can add to total energy expenditure, just like structured exercise. This is why it's better for your metabolism if you avoid sitting for long periods of time & instead stay active all day long. Metabolic rate is affected by dietary factors as well. The fuel for your body's energy production comes from the foods you eat, & the kind of foods you eat can affect your metabolic rate. The amount of energy needed for food digestion, absorption, & metabolism is called the thermic effect of food (TEF). Thermic effects of various macronutrients (proteins, carbs, & fats) vary. One example is protein; unlike carbs & fats, it has a greater thermic effect, which means that the body expends more energy digesting protein-rich meals. Muscle mass preservation, which is inversely proportional to metabolic rate, is another critical function of protein. Conversely, carbohydrates offer a rapid energy boost, but too much of them, particularly refined carbs & sugars, which lead to increases in blood glucose levels &, consequently, weight gain. When consumed in moderation, healthy fats—like the monounsaturated fats & omega-3 fatty acids included in foods like nuts, fatty fish, olive oil, & oil have a greater energy density & can help the metabolism work more efficiently. The metabolic dysfunction, obesity, & insulin resistance that can result from eating too many bad fats, like trans fats, is real. Metabolic function is dependent on both macronutrients & micronutrients, such as vitamins & minerals. Some examples of essential nutrients include magnesium, which plays a role in muscle function & insulin sensitivity, & the B vitamins, which are essential for energy production. Inadequate intake of iron, iodine, & zinc can cause metabolic imbalances & exhaustion, all of which are detrimental to a healthy metabolism. An essential part of metabolism is the regulation of hormones. Almost every metabolic process in the body is impacted by hormones, which are chemical messengers. Hormones control energy production, fat storage, & hunger. Thyroid hormones (T3 & T4), alongside insulin, leptin, ghrelin, cortisol, & growth hormone, are important hormones that impact metabolism. An essential function of thyroid hormones is to control the resting metabolic rate of the body. Hypothyroidism is characterized by low thyroid hormone levels, which cause a slowdown in metabolism & a host of symptoms including increased appetite, lethargy, & intolerance to cold. When the thyroid is overactive, a condition known as hyperthyroidism, the metabolism speeds up, which in turn can cause anxiety, rapid heartbeat, & weight loss. One of the most important functions of the pancreatic hormone insulin is to control blood sugar levels & to store energy. Insulin resistance is a metabolic disorder characterized by impaired insulin action & elevated blood sugar levels; it is common in people who are overweight or have type 2 diabetes. The hormones leptin & ghrelin control food intake. The hormone leptin is secreted by adipose tissue & tells the brain that there is sufficient energy in the body to quell hunger. In contrast, the stomach secretes ghrelin, which triggers hunger pangs. Overeating & excess weight gain can result from hormonal imbalances. In times of chronic stress, the stress hormone cortisol can also impact metabolism by increasing hunger & promoting fat storage. A key player in controlling fat metabolism & keeping muscle mass intact is growth hormone, which is secreted by the pituitary gland. A person's metabolic rate is also affected by how much sleep they get. Insulin resistance, increased hunger, & changes in glucose processing are metabolic disturbances that can result from insufficient or poor sleep. An increase in cravings for high-calorie foods & overeating can be attributed to sleep deprivation, which raises levels of the hunger hormone ghrelin & lowers levels of the satiety hormone leptin. Circadian rhythms govern the body's inherent sleep-wake cycle & impact metabolic functions; insomnia can throw these rhythms out of whack. Weight gain & metabolic diseases like type 2 diabetes & obesity can be exacerbated by chronic sleep deprivation. Metabolic rate is also greatly affected by stress. Elevated cortisol levels, brought on by persistent stress, encourage fat storage, especially in the abdominal region. Hormones that control hunger, such as leptin & ghrelin, are impacted by stress, which causes an increase in hunger & a desire for unhealthy food. In addition to having a negative impact on metabolism already, stress can make it even harder to sleep. Temperature & exposure to pollutants are two examples of environmental variables that can affect metabolic function. As an example, brown adipose tissue (BAT)—a sort of fat that burns calories to produce heat—can be activated by cold exposure, which can increase energy expenditure. Conversely, environmental pollutants, such as endocrine disruptors in plastics, can cause metabolic disorders &

weight gain by interfering with hormone regulation. Age, gender, heredity, muscular mass, exercise, nutrition, hormonal control, stress, & environmental exposures are just a few of the many factors that impact metabolism. When it comes to energy metabolism, hormone regulation, & general health, each of these factors is important in its own way. To optimize metabolism, improve energy balance, & reduce the risk of metabolic diseases, individuals must understand the complex interactions between these factors in order to make informed choices. Keeping metabolic health & promoting long-term wellness requires a combination of measures, including regular exercise, a balanced diet, stress management, sufficient sleep, & avoiding environmental pollutants.

The Role of Nutrition in Metabolism

A proper diet supplies the body with the building blocks for metabolism, which in turn regulates hormone levels, repairs damaged tissues, & produces energy. Micronutrient quality (vitamins & minerals), macronutrient balance (carbs, proteins, & fats), & the kinds of food we consume all play a role in how well our metabolism works. While a well-balanced, nutrient-rich diet promotes optimal metabolic function, unhealthy eating habits can cause metabolic imbalances, which in turn can cause insulin resistance, excess weight gain, diabetes, & heart disease. The body's energy & the maintenance of many metabolic processes are provided by the three primary macronutrients: carbohydrates, proteins, & fats. Cells use glucose, a byproduct of carbohydrate metabolism, for immediate energy needs or store it as glycogen in the liver & muscles for later use. How rapidly carbs are digested & absorbed into the bloodstream is affected by their glycemic index (GI). Refined sugars, white bread, & other foods with a high glycemic index (GI) raise insulin production because they cause blood sugar levels to spike quickly. Insulin resistance, a risk factor for metabolic syndrome & type 2 diabetes, can develop with time in a diet heavy in refined carbs. Whole grains, veggies, & legumes are good sources of low-GI carbohydrates because they are slowly digested, which means that they provide a steady release of glucose & help maintain more consistent energy levels throughout the day. Although carbs are a better source of immediate energy, fats are required for insulation, long-term energy storage, & hormone production. A person's metabolic health is greatly affected by the kind of fat they eat. Olive oil, avocados, & fatty fish are good sources of unsaturated fats, which help the metabolism work properly by decreasing inflammation, making the body more insulin sensitive, & increasing the rate at which fat is burned off. By improving mitochondrial function & decreasing fat accumulation, omega-3 fatty acids in particular have been demonstrated to lower the risk of metabolic diseases. Processed foods are a major source of trans fats & saturated fats, which are known to have negative effects on insulin function, inflammation, & metabolic dysfunction. In order to keep muscle mass, repair tissues, & support metabolic processes, protein is an essential macronutrient. Consumption of protein results in its breakdown into amino acids. These building blocks are then utilized to construct new proteins & provide support for the activity of enzymes, such as those involved in nutrient metabolism & energy production. Because muscle tissue burns more calories at rest than fat tissue, a higher metabolic rate is directly correlated with maintaining muscle mass, which can be achieved by consuming an adequate amount of protein. The energy needed to digest, absorb, & metabolize nutrients—the thermic effect of food (TEF)—increases with increasing protein consumption. The thermogenesis of food containing protein is greater than that of food containing carbs or fats because protein has a higher thermogenesis factor (TEF). Protein also aids in appetite regulation by decreasing hunger pangs & increasing satiety, which in turn makes it easier to control weight & maintain metabolic balance. Vitamins, minerals, & antioxidants are examples of micronutrients that are just as important for metabolism regulation as macronutrients. To produce energy & carry out the metabolism of carbs, lipids, & proteins, the body requires the B vitamins, which include B1 (thiamine), B2 (riboflavin), B3 (niacin), B5 (pantothenic acid), B6 (pyridoxine), B7 (biotin), B9 (folic acid), & B12 (cobalamin). In metabolic pathways, these vitamins work as coenzymes to help turn food into energy. For instance, the mitochondria, which are cellular organelles responsible for producing energy, cannot function properly without B12. Weak energy production, a sluggish metabolism, & lethargy are all symptoms of a B vitamin deficiency. Another crucial mineral for metabolic function, iron allows the blood to carry oxygen. Adequate iron levels are critical for sustaining energy levels & cellular respiration; hemoglobin, a protein in red blood cells that transports oxygen to tissues, contains iron. The body uses magnesium to support more than 300 enzyme reactions, including those that produce energy & function muscles, & zinc to regulate insulin & glucose metabolism. Sunlight triggers the skin to produce vitamin D, which is essential for metabolic health because it supports the immune system & affects insulin function. Insulin resistance, obesity, & metabolic diseases are all linked to insufficient vitamin D levels. Vitamins C & E, along with selenium & polyphenols in green tea, fruits, & vegetables all contain antioxidant properties that help shield cells from oxidative stress. This stress can harm tissues &

interfere with metabolic functions. The imbalance between antioxidants & free radicals causes oxidative stress, which in turn causes inflammation & metabolic dysfunction. To keep your metabolism in check & free radicals at bay, eat lots of fruits, vegetables, & whole foods. A healthy metabolism also benefits from fiber, another essential dietary component. Even though the body doesn't digest fiber directly, it helps with digestion, regulates blood sugar levels, & makes you feel full. Oats, beans, & fruits are good sources of soluble fiber, which helps control blood sugar levels by forming a gel-like substance in the digestive tract. This can help keep blood sugar levels steady all day long & avoid insulin spikes. Whole grains, veggies, & seeds are good sources of insoluble fiber, which aids digestion by adding bulk to stool & encouraging regular bowel movements. Reduced risk of metabolic diseases like type 2 diabetes & cardiovascular disease has also been associated with fiber-rich diets. This is because fiber aids in cholesterol regulation, insulin sensitivity improvement, & weight maintenance. One of the most underrated dietary components that has a major impact on metabolic rate is hydration. Almost every metabolic process relies on water, including nutrient absorption, temperature regulation, & waste product elimination. In addition to lowering energy levels & slowing digestion, dehydration can hinder metabolic function, which in turn causes lethargy & weariness. Because glucose & other nutrients must be transported to cells by water, an inadequate water intake can also impact the body's capacity to control blood sugar levels. Maintaining a healthy metabolism & optimal energy levels can be achieved by drinking water regularly throughout the day. Another factor that can affect metabolism is the timing & frequency of meals. Blood sugar levels can be stabilized & energy crashes prevented by eating small, balanced meals throughout the day. When you go for long periods without eating, your metabolism slows down because your body goes into conservation mode, which means it burns less energy & less fat. Supporting weight management & metabolic health, a well-balanced diet rich in protein, healthy fats, & fiber can regulate hunger hormones & curb overeating. Furthermore, new studies have demonstrated that a metabolic boost, improved insulin sensitivity, & enhanced cellular repair processes can be achieved through intermittent fasting, a type of eating & fasting that alternates between periods of eating & not eating. Nevertheless, variables like age, gender, & general health can affect how well intermittent fasting works for different people. Caffeine is another food that can speed up your metabolism for a short while. Caffeine is a stimulant that can increase metabolic rate & energy expenditure; it is present in coffee, tea, & some energy drinks. Although the effects of caffeine on resting metabolic rate tend to diminish with regular consumption owing to tolerance, studies have demonstrated that it can increase the rate by up to 5%. While a moderate amount of caffeine can help the metabolism work, too much of it can cause problems like racing thoughts, anxiety, & insomnia. Metabolic support through a balanced, nutrient-rich diet prioritizes natural, unprocessed foods that are rich in fiber, micronutrients, & macronutrients. Metabolic optimization, energy balance, & metabolic disorder prevention are all possible when people eat a diet high in foods that support cellular function, hormone regulation, & energy production. Metabolic function can be further improved by hydration, meal timing, & certain dietary patterns such as intermittent fasting, in addition to macronutrients & micronutrients. A healthy metabolism & long-term health goals can be achieved through mindful eating, an emphasis on nutrient-dense foods, regular exercise, stress management, & sufficient sleep.

Macronutrients & Their Impact on Energy

The three macronutrients—carbohydrates, proteins, & fats—are the building blocks of all of the energy that the human body needs to perform its many metabolic functions, including maintaining & enhancing growth, development, & health. If you want to eat healthily, perform at your best, control your weight, & optimize your performance in physical activities, you must know how these macronutrients influence energy production & metabolism. Due to their high energy density & ease of breakdown into glucose, the body's primary fuel for cells, tissues, & organs, carbohydrates rank high among the most efficient & immediate sources of energy the body has. When you exercise, your brain & muscles use the simple sugar glucose for fuel. This sugar is always present in your bloodstream. Complex carbohydrates, such as starches, are broken down into glucose molecules in the small intestine as part of the digestion process that starts in the mouth. Fruits, vegetables, & dairy products are good sources of simple carbohydrates, which are sugars that the body can absorb easily. But refined carbs like white bread, pasta, & sugary snacks raise insulin & blood sugar levels quickly, which causes energy crashes &, in the long run, insulin resistance. Glycogen stores carbohydrates in the liver & muscles; when blood glucose levels drop or during intense physical activity, the body can draw on these stores. People are able to keep going for long periods of time because glycogen is a readily available energy reserve. In order to maximize performance & avoid fatigue, athletes & active people prioritize carbohydrate intake. This is because the body prefers carbohydrates as a fuel source. Having said that, the effect of carbs on energy levels varies widely. Whole grains, legumes, & vegetables are good sources of complex carbs because they take longer to digest & release glucose into the bloodstream. This means that you can eat them for sustained energy without worrying about the wild swings in your blood sugar levels that simple sugars cause. A high fiber content is another benefit of these complex carbohydrates; it helps with digestion, promotes good gut health, & keeps blood sugar levels stable. A healthy, balanced diet must include complex carbs because they are essential for energy & because fiber makes you feel full for longer, which helps you control your portion sizes & maintain a healthy weight. Carbohydrates are essential for energy metabolism, but fats are even more important for producing energy over the long term & storing calories. Carbohydrates provide short-term energy spikes, but fats are better for sustained energy because of their density & efficiency. Calories per gram of fat are more than double those of carbs & proteins, making fats an extremely energy dense food choice. When carbohydrate reserves are low or during long periods of moderate-intensity exercise, the body can use the energy produced by breaking down fats into fatty acids & glycerol. When energy needs are met, fats stored in adipose tissue are released into the bloodstream. Lipolysis is the breakdown of lipids into their component energy molecules. This process occurs in the mitochondria of cells, which are commonly called the body's powerhouses. Factors including metabolic flexibility, amount of physical activity, & dietary composition affect the body's ability to convert fat into energy efficiently. During periods of calorie restriction or endurance exercise, the body switches from using carbs as an energy source to using fat stores. This is why fat is the main fuel source for long-duration activities like marathons or long bike rides. Omega-3 & omega-6 fatty acids, which are present in healthy fats like avocados, nuts, seeds, & fatty fish, are crucial for lowering inflammation, bolstering brain function, & keeping the heart healthy. As an added bonus, these fats help regulate hormone production & help the body absorb fat-soluble vitamins (A, D, E, & K). Metabolic dysfunction, insulin resistance, & an elevated risk of cardiovascular diseases can result from eating an excessive quantity of saturated fats found in processed foods or trans fats. For a healthy metabolism & balanced energy intake, it's best to eat fats moderately, preferably unsaturated fats derived from whole foods. Although protein is most commonly linked to constructing & repairing muscles, it is also essential for energy metabolism. Although the body does not rely on protein as its principal fuel source, it is necessary for the development & maintenance of tissues, such as muscles, & can serve as an alternative energy source in the absence of carbs & fats. Proteins can be broken down into amino acids & converted into glucose through a process called gluconeogenesis during periods of intense physical activity or prolonged fasting. Even when glycogen stores are low, the body is able to keep blood glucose levels stable & keep the brain & muscles powered. Protein doesn't play a huge role in the body's energy production compared to carbs & fats, but getting enough protein is still important for maintaining muscle mass & a healthy metabolism. A steady supply of amino acids is essential for the structure & function of muscles, which are metabolically active tissues. Hence, protein aids in the maintenance of muscle mass, which is positively associated with a higher metabolic rate, & thus plays an indirect role in metabolism. A higher resting metabolic rate (RMR) indicates that an individual burns more calories at rest when they have more muscle mass. Because of this, eating a lot of high-quality protein can aid with weight management & keep muscles from getting weak, particularly as we get older or lose weight. It takes more energy for the body to digest, absorb, & metabolize protein-rich meals than it does for carbs & fats because protein has a greater thermic effect. Total energy expenditure & metabolic function are both aided by this food's thermic effect (TEF). A more metabolically demanding macronutrient than carbs & lipids, protein has a TEF of 20-30% compared to 5-10% for carbs & 0-3% for lipids. Additionally, protein aids in weight management by reducing hunger & increasing control over appetite. The regulation of energy production, metabolism, & general health are all affected by the dietary balance of carbs, fats, & proteins. When broken down into their component parts, macronutrients provide the building blocks the body needs for energy production, fuel storage, & tissue repair, among other vital functions. Consuming a balanced macronutrient diet & making smart food choices that promote metabolic efficiency are the two most important factors in maintaining a healthy metabolism. To aid in energy production, stabilize blood sugar levels, & lower the risk of metabolic disorders, one needs a diet abundant in whole grains, lean proteins, healthy fats, fruits, veggies, & legumes. The body's capacity to process macronutrients & produce energy is further improved by adequate hydration, micronutrient consumption, & sleep. In order to maximize energy expenditure, enhance metabolic health, & contribute to general well-being, it is recommended to combine a balanced diet with regular physical activity.

Metabolism-Boosting Foods & Nutrients

To improve energy production, control weight, & keep one's health in check, one must eat foods & take nutrients that boost metabolism. Although factors like heredity, age, &

exercise level do have an impact on metabolism, certain nutrients & foods can aid metabolic processes, boost energy expenditure, & reduce the risk of metabolic disorders. By improving insulin sensitivity, speeding up fat burning, & increasing thermogenesis (the body's heat production process), these nutrients & foods can help improve metabolic efficiency.

Epigallocatechin gallate (EGCG), an antioxidant found in green tea, is one of the most famous foods that stimulates the metabolism. Catechins are powerful antioxidants that have been proven to enhance fat oxidation & energy expenditure. Researchers have shown that green tea extract can make you burn more calories even when you're not moving around. Additionally, green tea has caffeine, which can increase metabolic rate (particularly when coupled with exercise) by stimulating the central nervous system. Coffee, tea, & even some energy drinks contain caffeine, a stimulant. Its capacity to raise metabolic rate & fat oxidation has been known for some time. Caffeine, by triggering the secretion of adrenaline, aids in the breakdown of adipose tissue into usable free fatty acids. It is important to consume caffeine moderately because its effects on metabolism may diminish with regular consumption owing to tolerance.

Protein, especially from high-quality sources such as lean meats, seafood, eggs, beans, & dairy products, is another powerful nutrient that boosts metabolism. Thermic effect of food (TEF) calculations show that the digestion, absorption, & processing of protein requires more energy than those of carbs & lipids. Total daily calorie expenditure rises as a result of this. The resting metabolic rate (RMR) is increased by protein because it aids in muscle maintenance & growth. A person's basal metabolic rate (BMR) is directly proportional to the amount of muscle mass they have, since the metabolic activity of muscles is greater than that of fat. Eating foods high in protein can aid with weight management by reducing hunger pangs & making you feel full on fewer calories.

It is well-known that spicy foods, especially those with capsaicin (the active ingredient in chili peppers), can momentarily increase metabolic rate. Capsaicin boosts thermogenesis, which in turn increases calorie burning & promotes fat release from fat cells. Consuming spicy foods may enhance caloric expenditure by approximately 8% for a period of thirty minutes following consumption, according to research. When coupled with exercise, this effect may enhance fat burning, making it an ideal choice for those looking to maximize their workout benefits. Spicy foods can be a useful addition to a diet that aims to boost metabolism, even though the effects are temporary.

The metabolism benefits from the complex carbs & fiber found in whole grains such as oats, quinoa, brown rice, & barley. In order to keep blood sugar levels stable & avoid insulin spikes, which can cause fat storage, whole grains are a good source of fiber. In addition to lowering hunger & aiding in calorie control, fiber promotes fullness. In addition, the digestive process of whole grains uses more energy than that of refined grains, so eating more whole grains can help you burn more calories. Unlike refined grains & processed sugars, which cause blood sugar crashes, whole grains' carbs are slowly digested & absorbed, providing a steady supply of glucose for energy.

One more food that can help the metabolism work better is coconut oil, which has medium-chain triglycerides (MCTs). Monounsaturated fatty acids (MCTs) are metabolized differently than the long-chain fatty acids (LCFAs) present in the majority of oils. The liver converts MCTs into energy more quickly, which aids in fat burning. Increasing calorie burning & decreasing body fat may be possible with MCT consumption, according to some research. Coconut oil is an excellent choice for individuals wishing to enhance their metabolism & aid in weight loss because medium-chain triglycerides (MCTs) are not as readily stored as other forms of fat. A fast & efficient way to boost energy & aid in fat loss is to add coconut oil to your meals or smoothies.

There are many health benefits to consuming small amounts of apple cider vinegar (ACV), one of which is supporting metabolic health. Research has shown that the acetic acid in ACV can help regulate blood sugar levels & increase insulin sensitivity. The body may be able to process & store glucose more effectively with the help of ACV, which improves insulin sensitivity. This could help prevent fat accumulation & support healthy weight management. You can cut back on calories by using apple cider vinegar to curb your hunger & make you feel full faster. Moderate use of apple cider vinegar (ACV) can complement a healthy diet, but further study is required to determine its long-term effects on metabolism.

A healthy metabolism can benefit from the antioxidants, fiber, & vitamins found in berries like strawberries, blueberries, & raspberries. Polyphenols are plant compounds that have anti-inflammatory & insulin-stimulating properties; berries contain a disproportionately high amount of these compounds. Reducing inflammation can help optimize metabolic function, as it is linked to metabolic disorders like obesity & diabetes. Berries are a metabolic booster due to their high fiber content, which aids in sugar regulation & bowel health. Berry consumption also prevents rapid increases in blood sugar levels due to their low glycemic index (GI).

Consuming leafy greens such as spinach, kale, & Swiss chard can help support a healthy metabolism & general well-being. Magnesium, which is abundant in these foods, is essential for the proper functioning of muscles & more than 300 other biochemical reactions in the body. In addition to its role in insulin function & blood sugar regulation, magnesium is essential for the proper contraction & relaxation of muscles, which in turn helps to keep muscle mass & metabolic rate stable. In addition to providing the necessary vitamins & minerals to optimize metabolism, the low calorie content of leafy greens makes them a great option for individuals trying to control their weight.

Almonds, walnuts, chia seeds, flaxseeds, & other nuts & seeds are great for boosting metabolism because they are rich in healthy fats, protein, & fiber. All three of these macronutrients work together in nuts & seeds to make you feel full faster, keep your blood sugar steady, & burn more calories. A diet high in nuts, especially walnuts & almonds, can help lower the risk of metabolic diseases like type 2 diabetes & cardiovascular disease due to the anti-inflammatory characteristics of omega-3 fatty acids. In addition to promoting good digestion & aiding in appetite regulation, the high fiber content of nuts & seeds can help you maintain a healthy weight.

Although it is not technically a food, water is a necessary component for all of the body's metabolic processes. Nutrient absorption, energy production, & waste elimination all rely on water, so it's crucial to stay hydrated for optimal metabolic function. Metabolic rate slowdown, energy loss, & impaired physical performance are all symptoms of dehydration. Additionally, drinking water before meals can aid with appetite control by making you feel full faster, which may cause you to eat less calories overall. Because it takes energy to bring cold water to body temperature, drinking it can slightly boost metabolism.

Lastly, the probiotics found in fermented foods such as kimchi, sauerkraut, yogurt, & kefir help keep the digestive tract healthy. Digestive health, nutrient absorption, & metabolic process regulation all depend on a balanced gut microbiome. Obesity & insulin resistance are metabolic disorders that have been linked to a disruption in the normal balance of gut bacteria. In addition to promoting a healthier metabolism & decreasing inflammation, fermented foods aid in restoring balance to the gut microbiota. In addition to improving metabolic efficiency, eating foods rich in probiotics on a regular basis can boost the body's nutrient processing & utilization abilities.

A healthy metabolism is essential for energy production, blood sugar regulation, fat burning, & overall wellness, & these foods & nutrients can help you achieve just that with a well-rounded diet. Although there is no one food or nutrient that can magically make you lose weight or speed up your metabolism, eating a variety of these foods can have a multiplicative effect on your metabolism, energy expenditure, & overall health.

Common Dietary Mistakes That Slow Metabolism

The complex process of metabolism involves converting food into energy. While factors like age, genetics, & physical activity can affect metabolic rate, a person's diet has a major impact on how efficiently the body burns calories & uses nutrients. Unwanted weight gain, low energy, & an increased risk of metabolic diseases like diabetes, obesity, & insulin resistance can result from some food habits. In order to support metabolic health & maintain an optimal weight, it is important to understand these common dietary mistakes. By doing so, individuals can make better food choices.

1. Not Eating Enough Calories or Skipping Meals

Skipping meals or drastically cutting calories is a common but disastrous diet mistake. Losing weight by cutting calories may sound like a no-brainer, but doing so repeatedly puts the body into "starvation mode." Calories burned per day are reduced as the body slows down its metabolism to conserve energy. Loss of muscle mass, a slowed metabolic rate, & diminished energy levels are all possible outcomes of not getting enough nutrients when you skip meals. To keep metabolism running smoothly & provide energy for the body, it's important to eat a balanced diet high in nutrient-dense foods.

2. Consuming Foods That Have Been Processed or Refined

Metabolic rate can be drastically reduced by consuming an abundance of processed & refined foods, including sugary snacks, baked products, & fast food. The unhealthy fats, sugars, & simple carbs found in these foods can trigger rapid increases & decreases in blood sugar, leaving you feeling tired & hungry. In the long run, eating these foods can make your body less effective at regulating your blood sugar levels through insulin. Insulin resistance is associated with a slowed metabolism & an increase in body fat, especially in the abdominal region. For a healthy metabolism, it's best to avoid processed foods & instead eat whole, nutrient-dense foods like fruits, vegetables, lean meats, whole grains, & healthy fats.

3. Excessive Sugar Consumption

Consuming an excessive amount of sugar, particularly refined sugars & sugary drinks, can hinder metabolism. Blood glucose levels rise in response to a high-sugar diet, which in turn causes the body to secrete insulin. But insulin resistance develops when blood sugar levels stay high for an extended period of time as a result of chronically high sugar intake, & this hinders the body's capacity to metabolize nutrients efficiently. Insulin resistance raises the risk of metabolic diseases such as obesity & type 2 diabetes & slows the metabolism. If you want to improve insulin sensitivity, support a healthy metabolism, & lower your risk of weight gain, cut back on sugary foods & drinks.

4. Eating Too Much Processed Fats

Fats are a macronutrient that the body needs for energy, hormone production, & the absorption of vitamins that are fat-soluble. However, not all fats are the same. Metabolic function can be impaired by eating a diet rich in unhealthy fats, especially trans fats & an excess of saturated fats. Particularly dangerous are trans fats, which are present in processed foods such as baked goods, snacks, & margarine. These fats can enhance inflammation, impair insulin sensitivity, & encourage fat storage. Although saturated fats are not as bad for you as trans fats, eating too much of them can still make you put on weight & slow down your metabolism. Olive oil, avocado, nuts, seeds, & fatty fish are good sources of unsaturated fats, which are better for you because they support a healthy metabolism & lower inflammation.

5. Protein Insufficiency

Tissue formation & repair, muscle maintenance, & metabolic support all rely on protein. A lack of protein in the diet is a common mistake that many people make, & it can cause them to gradually lose muscle mass. The metabolic rate of muscle tissue is higher than that of fat tissue, even when at rest. It becomes more challenging to maintain a healthy weight when muscle mass decreases as a result of inadequate protein consumption, as this slows down the metabolism. Protein also has a greater thermic effect of food (TEF) than fats & carbs, which means that the digestion & processing of protein-rich foods requires more energy from the body. Supporting muscle maintenance & boosting metabolism requires an adequate intake of high-quality protein sources like lean meats, poultry, fish, legumes, & dairy.

6. Consumption of Inadequate Water

A person's metabolic rate can be drastically affected by dehydration. The digestive process, the absorption of nutrients, & the proper operation of metabolic processes all rely on water. A slowed metabolism, less energy, & worse performance in physical activities are all symptoms of dehydration. Because it takes energy to bring water to body temperature, drinking cold water, in particular, can boost metabolism by roughly 30% for as little as 30 minutes, according to some studies. Furthermore, dehydration can trigger hunger pangs, which in turn can lead to overeating & thwart attempts at weight loss. Staying hydrated all day long with water & water-rich foods like veggies & fruits is crucial for supporting optimal metabolic function.

Avoiding Carbohydrates That Are Good For You

Although carbohydrates are frequently vilified in diets aimed at weight loss, they really serve as the body's primary fuel source. Selecting appropriate carbs is crucial. In the long term, your metabolism might suffer if you cut out healthy, complex carbs or completely avoid carbs. Legumes, fruits, vegetables, & whole grains all contain a lot of fiber, which helps to stabilize blood sugar levels & prevent insulin spikes by slowly releasing glucose into the bloodstream. Additionally, these foods help you feel full for longer, which means you can better manage your hunger & avoid eating too much. However, nutrient deficits, exhaustion, & a slowed metabolism can emerge from relying on low-carb or no-carb diets that limit these beneficial energy sources.

8. Excessive Salt Consumption

Water retention & elevated blood pressure, brought on by an excess of sodium in the diet, have a deleterious effect on metabolism, putting a strain on the cardiovascular system & lowering energy levels generally. Feeling lethargic & bloated are symptoms of water retention, which can occur when salt consumption is high. In addition to making it harder to stick to a balanced diet & keep a healthy metabolism, a high-salt diet can increase cravings for unhealthy foods. To aid with weight loss & metabolic health, cut back on processed foods, canned soups, & salty snacks to lower sodium intake.

9. The Problem of Varying Meal Times

The circadian rhythm controls metabolism & is activated when eating habits are irregular. Disrupting the body's ability to efficiently process food & burn calories can be achieved by eating at inconsistent times or having long periods of fasting followed by large meals. Optimal metabolic function & better weight management can be achieved by eating in harmony with the body's natural circadian rhythm, which includes avoiding late-night eating & eating at regular intervals throughout the day. Regular, well-balanced meals & snacks eaten at regular intervals throughout the day can aid in metabolic health & blood sugar regulation.

10. Excessive Alcohol Consumption

Drinking too much alcohol can impair the body's fat-burning mechanisms & slow down the metabolism. Fat oxidation & energy expenditure are both slowed down when the body metabolizes alcohol because it takes precedence over other nutrients. Furthermore, alcohol contributes to weight gain due to its high calorie content & lack of nutritional value when consumed in excess. Consumption of alcohol on a regular basis has negative effects on hormone regulation & sleep quality, which in turn hinders metabolic function. Limiting alcohol consumption is important to prevent negative effects on metabolic health, even though moderate consumption may not significantly affect metabolism.

Exercise & Physical Activity

A healthy metabolism & the prevention of many chronic diseases depend on regular exercise & other forms of physical activity. Beyond the obvious effects on calorie expenditure during exercise, regular physical activity affects metabolic function generally, energy balance specifically, fat oxidation, muscle mass maintenance, & overall. Exercise has a direct impact on metabolic rate, which is the rate at which the body burns calories. This is because exercise increases muscle mass, improves cardiovascular health, & makes fat burning more efficient. Anyone can optimize their physical activity routines to improve metabolic function & overall well-being by understanding the role of exercise in metabolism & how different types of exercise contribute to energy health.

The Effects of Different Exercises on Metabolism:

Exercise, specifically aerobic exercise, strength training, & high-intensity interval training (HIIT), has a profound effect on metabolism. The metabolic rate & energy levels can be enhanced through a variety of exercises, each of which has its own special advantages.

Aerobic exercise raises the heart rate & oxygen consumption; examples of aerobic exercise include walking, jogging, swimming, cycling, & dancing. This form of exercise improves cardiovascular health, burns calories, & enhances fat oxidation by primarily using carbs & fat as fuel. When you engage in aerobic exercise, particularly for extended periods of moderate activity, your body's ability to burn fat for energy is enhanced. Aerobic exercise improves endurance & calorie expenditure during & after exercise by increasing the efficiency of mitochondria, the cells' energy-producing powerhouses. This effect is maintained over time with regular aerobic exercise. Improved insulin sensitivity, brought about by aerobic exercise, aids in blood sugar regulation & wards off insulin resistance.

Resistance training, often known as strength training, aims to increase bone density & muscle mass via the use of weightlifting & resistance bands. Because of its higher metabolic rate, muscle tissue has a higher energy maintenance requirement than adipose tissue. The amount of calories burned while at rest, or resting metabolic rate (RMR), can be increased by strengthening one's muscles. In addition to preserving lean tissue & slowing the metabolic rate drop that comes with getting older, strength training is essential for avoiding muscle loss as people get older. Strength training not only helps you gain muscle, but it also makes you stronger overall, which means you can move around more efficiently when you need to. It also improves your muscular endurance & joint health.

High-Intensity Interval Training (HIIT): In HIIT, you work out at a high level for short intervals of time before recovering or reducing the intensity. Its rapid metabolic elevation & time-efficiency have contributed to its meteoric rise in popularity as an exercise modality. The term "post-exercise oxygen consumption" (EPOC) refers to the fact that your body keeps burning calories even when you're not moving, & research has demonstrated that HIIT increases this rate. The "afterburn effect" can continue for a few more hours, adding to your total caloric expenditure. In particular, high-intensity interval training (HIIT) boosts metabolic flexibility, which allows the body to use a variety of fuel sources (including carbs & fats) depending on its needs, & it improves cardiovascular health. High-intensity interval training (HIIT) boosts metabolic function, insulin sensitivity, & fat loss.

Muscle Mass & Its Impact on Metabolism:

Muscle mass is among the most influential variables on metabolic rate. Maintaining muscle mass demands more energy than maintaining fat mass because of the higher metabolic rate of muscle tissue. Consequently, a higher resting metabolic rate (RMR) indicates that the body burns more calories even when at rest, which can be achieved by exercising to increase muscle mass. The natural decline in muscle mass that comes with aging makes this all the more crucial, since it increases the likelihood of slowing the metabolism & putting on weight. When it comes to gaining & keeping muscle mass, strength training is your best bet, particularly as you get older. Muscle mass, when maintained or increased through aerobic exercise & strength training, supports a higher metabolic rate, lowers the risk of metabolic diseases & obesity, & helps people stay or look their best.

Metabolic Flexibility & Its Significance:

What we mean by metabolic flexibility is the body's capacity to use a variety of fuel sources, most commonly carbs & fats, depending on what's available & what the body needs. A person with metabolic flexibility can use fat for fuel efficiently when exercising or fasting at low intensities & carbs for quick energy when exercising at high intensities. Exercising regularly, especially with aerobic & HIIT forms of exercise, trains the body to use fat more efficiently & switch between fuel sources more effectively, which improves metabolic flexibility. An important part of metabolic health is improved metabolic flexibility, which is linked to better insulin sensitivity, less fat storage, & increased fat burning ability.

Insulin Sensitivity & Physical Activity:

Improving insulin sensitivity is one of the main advantages of exercising regularly. A hormone called insulin aids in glucose uptake into cells for energy, which in turn helps to control blood sugar levels. Metabolic diseases like type 2 diabetes are characterized by insulin resistance, which makes glucose processing more difficult & ultimately causes increased fat storage & high blood sugar levels. Exercising aerobically & strength training both increase insulin sensitivity, which in turn improves glucose processing & lowers the risk of metabolic diseases. Exercising improves insulin sensitivity, which in turn aids in glucose regulation, fat oxidation, & metabolic health in general.

Fat Loss & Exercise:

Maintaining a healthy metabolic rate requires a reduction in body fat, which is best accomplished through consistent physical activity. By raising the metabolic rate, increasing the amount of calories burned, & enhancing fat oxidation, high-intensity interval training (HIIT), strength training, & aerobic exercise all aid in fat loss. Because it improves metabolic flexibility & increases post-exercise calorie burning, HIIT in particular is very effective for fat loss. Raising your resting metabolic rate & encouraging fat burning while you're at rest are two of the many ways in which strength training contributes to your fat loss efforts. For optimal metabolic health & fat loss, it is best to combine aerobic exercise with strength training or high-intensity interval training (HIIT).

Physical Activity & Hormonal Balance:

Regulating hormones that impact metabolism is another important function of exercise. Hormones like leptin, ghrelin, insulin, & cortisol all have a part in controlling hunger, fat storage, & energy expenditure; physical exercise helps keep these hormones in check. Exercising regularly lowers cortisol levels, which in turn lower chronic stress & its associated increases in fat storage, especially in the abdominal region. Exercise promotes a more efficient metabolism, lowers the risk of metabolic diseases & obesity by lowering stress levels & improving hormonal balance. Exercising also aids in the regulation of hunger hormones such as leptin & ghrelin, which in turn promotes improved appetite control & decreases the probability of overeating.

Effects of Physical Activity on Emotional Well-Being & Drive:

In addition to the obvious physical benefits, regular exercise also has important psychological advantages that contribute to better metabolic health in the long run. Engaging in regular physical activity has a positive impact on mood by releasing endorphins, which are neurotransmitters that alleviate anxiety & depression. When people feel better emotionally & mentally, they are more likely to be motivated to lead active lives & eat healthily, which is good for their metabolism. To top it all off, a healthy metabolism relies on good sleep, which can be enhanced with regular exercise. Physical & mental well-being are enhanced through exercise, which is especially important because insufficient sleep is associated with metabolic dysfunction, which includes insulin resistance, increased hunger, & weight gain.

Integrating Physical Activity into Everyday Routines:

To keep metabolic health, it's necessary to engage in physical activity on a daily basis in addition to following a structured exercise program. Increase your daily calorie expenditure & improve your metabolic health with simple changes like taking the stairs instead of the elevator, walking or biking to work, or engaging in recreational activities. Keeping moving at regular intervals throughout the day will help you burn more calories & keep your metabolism going strong. Exercise is more likely to become a sustainable & pleasurable part of daily life if you incorporate it into activities that you enjoy & that bring you joy.

How Exercise Affects Metabolism

Metabolic rate, the rate at which the body uses food for energy, is significantly affected by exercise. When we work out, our muscles, organs, & tissues use more energy, so these processes speed up to keep up. Nevertheless, the metabolic benefits of exercise go beyond just burning calories in the short term. By keeping up with a regular exercise routine, you can improve your metabolic efficiency, raise your resting metabolic rate (RMR), & alter your body's nutrient processing, energy balance regulation, & fat-burning abilities over time. Improving metabolic health through exercise requires an understanding of the effects of various forms of exercise on the metabolic rate.

One, You Burn More Calories When You Work Out

Calorie expenditure rises as a direct result of exercise, making it one of the metabolic benefits felt most quickly. It takes more energy to fuel muscle contractions, keep the body at a constant temperature, & support cardiovascular function when we exercise, especially when we engage big muscle groups, like when we run, swim, or ride a bike. The number of calories burned during exercise is directly proportional to its intensity & length. Exercising at a higher intensity, like jogging or HIIT, can increase calorie expenditure because it raises the heart rate & energy demands more work than, say, walking or yoga.

When you engage in aerobic activities like jogging, cycling, or swimming, your body uses oxygen more efficiently & stores energy mainly in the form of carbs & fat. Aerobic exercise increases calorie expenditure because the body gets better at using fat as fuel for longer periods of exercise. Because of this, aerobic exercise is a great option for increasing both total energy expenditure & the ability to burn fat.

While strength training (also known as resistance exercise) does have an immediate calorie-burning effect, its main impact on metabolism is more long-term. Strength training demands energy because it challenges muscles with weights or resistance bands, which promotes hypertrophy & protein synthesis in muscles. Strength training raises the resting metabolic rate (RMR) more than aerobic exercise does, even though the number of calories burned right away may be lower due to the relative inactivity of muscle & fat.

Step Two: Consumption of Oxygen After Exercise (EPOC)

The afterburn effect, or excess post-exercise oxygen consumption (EPOC), keeps the body burning calories at a higher rate for a while after exercise. During the recovery phase following strenuous physical exercise, this phenomenon manifests as an elevated metabolic rate & increased oxygen uptake. To get back to resting state, replenish oxygen levels, remove metabolic waste (like lactic acid), repair muscle tissue, & so on, the body needs more energy.

The intensity & length of the workout determine the size & length of EPOC. As an example, moderate-intensity aerobic exercises, such as steady-state jogging, tend to have less of an EPOC effect than high-intensity interval training (HIIT) & resistance training. Depending on the intensity of the workout, the duration of EPOC can range from a few hours to up to 24 hours. During this time, the body continues to burn extra calories even when at rest.

Since the body burns fat more efficiently during the recovery phase of high-intensity workouts, this afterburn effect contributes to both increased calorie expenditure & fat loss. Therefore, if you want to boost your metabolism & lose fat, HIIT & strength training are your best bets.

3. Reduced Fatigue & Increased Muscle Mass (RMR)

The influence on muscle mass from consistent exercise is one of the most important long-term effects. Muscle tissue has a higher metabolic rate than adipose tissue, which means it uses more energy to stay in good shape. Muscle mass increases a person's resting metabolic rate (RMR), which means that they burn more calories even when they're not moving around. Building muscle can help reverse the metabolic slowdown that comes with getting older, making this a must-do for anyone trying to keep or lose weight.

To increase one's muscular mass, strength training is the way to go. Strength training with weights, bodyweight exercises, or resistance bands can halt the natural decline in muscle mass that comes with getting older or not moving around much. The resting metabolic rate (RMR) rises in tandem with muscle mass, meaning that as muscle grows, the body burns more calories all day long. This increases the body's ability to lose fat & improves energy balance.

Muscle protein synthesis, which strength training stimulates, is critical for post-workout repair & the development of new muscle fibers. It takes more energy to repair muscle tissue, & more muscle tissue means you burn more calories even when you're not moving around.

4. Greater Metabolic Adaptability

The ability of the body to efficiently transition between different energy sources, such as carbohydrates & fats, in response to availability & activity demands is known as metabolic flexibility. When you exercise regularly, especially with aerobic exercises & HIIT, your metabolic flexibility increases. This means that your body can use fat for energy when you're at rest or doing low-intensity activities, & carbs when you're working out hard.

Being metabolically flexible allows one to more readily transition between fueling oneself with glucose (derived from carbs) & fatty acids (derived from fat). In particular, this skill aids the body's ability to burn fat for fuel during fasting or long periods of exercise, & it also aids in preventing the accumulation of excess fat stores. Insulin sensitivity, fat accumulation, & metabolic efficiency are all positively correlated with increased metabolic flexibility.

The ability to use fat stores as fuel is enhanced through aerobic exercise, which includes activities such as walking, jogging, or cycling. However, by increasing mitochondrial efficiency & enhancing the uptake & utilization of oxygen during exercise, HIIT improves the body's ability to burn both carbohydrates & fat. More fat loss & more endurance are the long-term effects of this.

5. Metabolism & Hormonal Control

In addition to its obvious metabolic effects, exercise is critical for hormone regulation. Hormones like growth hormone, insulin, ghrelin, leptin, cortisol, & others play a major role in controlling hunger, energy balance, & fat storage. By keeping these hormones in check, regular exercise aids in metabolic function & weight management.

Exercise has many metabolic benefits, but improving insulin sensitivity is crucial. A hormone called insulin aids in glucose uptake into cells for energy, which in turn helps to control blood sugar levels. Insulin resistance hinders metabolism & raises the risk of type 2 diabetes; regular aerobic exercise & strength training enhance insulin sensitivity, which in turn makes glucose processing easier & lowers the risk of insulin resistance.

Intense physical activity & strength training cause the release of growth hormone, a hormone that helps with fat burning, muscle repair, & metabolic function generally. Having more growth hormone in your system aids in promoting fat loss, keeping your metabolism healthy, & preserving your lean muscle mass.

The stress hormone cortisol can be better controlled with regular exercise. Although cortisol plays a crucial role in the body's stress response, it is worth noting that prolonged exposure to high levels of cortisol can cause weight gain, especially in the abdominal region. By lowering cortisol levels & chronic stress, regular exercise improves metabolic health, evens out fat distribution, & boosts overall well-being.

Physical activity also affects the hunger hormones ghrelin & leptin. Leptin indicates fullness, while ghrelin promotes hunger. In order to maintain a healthy weight & avoid metabolic disruption & weight gain, it is important to exercise regularly because it helps balance these hormones, which in turn improves appetite control & prevents overeating.

6. Working Out, Reducing Body Fat, & Overall Health

Even though exercise helps you lose fat all over, the changes it brings about in your body composition have a major impact on your metabolic health. The term "body composition" describes the split between a person's fat mass & their lean mass, which includes things like muscle & bone. Because it takes more energy to maintain muscle tissue than fat tissue, a lower body fat percentage & a higher mass of muscle are linked to better metabolic function.

To improve body composition, one must engage in aerobic exercise & strength training simultaneously. The former helps burn fat while the latter increases muscle mass. In instance, when trying to gain muscle or avoid losing it while losing weight, strength training is absolutely necessary. Keeping or gaining muscle mass aids in metabolic rate elevation & promotes sustained fat loss. Both the short-term calorie burn & the long-term improvement in fat oxidation are mechanisms through which aerobic exercise aids in fat loss.

7. The Metabolic Impact of Chronic Exercise Over Time

The metabolic benefits of regular exercise last long after a single session has ended. Maintaining an exercise routine over time boosts mitochondrial function, muscle mass, & fat oxidation. The body's ability to burn fat, control blood sugar, & keep energy levels stable are all improved by these alterations.

Muscle mass & mitochondrial efficiency both naturally decrease with age, which causes a slowdown in metabolism. But by keeping or gaining muscle, enhancing mitochondrial function, & encouraging fat loss, regular exercise can help mitigate these effects. Supporting a healthy metabolism & lowering the risk of metabolic diseases like type 2 diabetes, cardiovascular disease, & obesity can be achieved through a routine that includes aerobic exercise, strength training, & high-intensity interval training (HIIT).

Cardio vs. Strength Training: Which is Better?

How Effective Is Cardio vs. Strength Training?

For a long time, advocates of both cardiovascular exercise (cardio) & strength training (strength training) have argued over which is better for health, fitness, & weight loss. Both forms of exercise are beneficial to the body in their own ways & should be part of any comprehensive fitness program, but they are distinct from one another & may be more or less effective depending on the person's objectives. Before deciding, it's important to learn about the differences between the two types of exercise, how they influence the body's energy systems & metabolism, & how they can work together for the best results in terms of health & fitness.

Exercise for the Heart (Cardio)

Activities that increase the heart rate & improve the efficiency of the heart & lungs are grouped together as cardiovascular exercise, or simply cardio. This category includes activities such as running, cycling, swimming, walking, & dancing. Aerobic endurance, cardiovascular health, & fat-burning capacity are the main goals of cardio. Cardio is a great way to get your heart rate up, your blood pumping, & your stamina up. Because it requires more energy to complete the exercise, it is also great for losing weight & burning calories.

Cardio has many benefits, but one of the most important is calorie burning, which is why it's so important for losing weight & reducing fat. Cardio, whether it's HIIT or moderate-intensity steady-state cardio (like a long, slow jog), is a great way to burn calories, which is essential for losing weight. Because it increases post-exercise calorie burning through the afterburn effect (excess post-exercise oxygen consumption, or EPOC), high-intensity interval training (HIIT) is well-known for its superior fat-burning capabilities compared to conventional steady-state cardio.

Cardiovascular exercise is also essential for better lung & heart health. By fortifying the cardiovascular system, it enhances the heart's capacity to pump blood & supply muscles with oxygen. Improved oxygen exchange during exercise is another benefit of increasing lung capacity. The prevention of cardiovascular diseases, such as heart disease & stroke, is one of these long-term benefits. Improved insulin sensitivity is a key component in regulating blood sugar levels & warding off metabolic disorders like type 2 diabetes; aerobic activities like jogging & cycling have this effect.

Training for Strength

Weights, resistance bands, or even just your own body weight in exercises like lunges, squats, & push-ups are all part of strength training, also known as resistance training. Gaining muscle, enhancing strength & endurance, & protecting joints are the main goals of strength training. Strength training places an emphasis on building muscle & strength, as opposed to cardiovascular exercise, which mainly uses the heart & lungs for energy.

Strength training helps you gain lean muscle mass, which is one of its main advantages. The metabolic rate (RMR) is the rate at which the body burns calories while at rest; this is because muscle tissue is more metabolically active than fat tissue. Increasing muscle mass via resistance exercises raises the RMR. In the long run, this makes strength training an effective tool for losing fat & keeping the weight off. A person's calorie expenditure, even when at rest (such as when sleeping or sitting), is directly proportional to their muscle mass.

Bone density is an important factor to consider when aging, & strength training can help with that. Osteoporosis, a condition characterized by weakened bones, can be mitigated through weight-bearing exercises, which stimulate bone growth & help maintain skeletal strength. Strength training not only helps with functional strength, which makes daily tasks easier, but it also helps with posture & balance, which are vital for aging people to avoid falls & injuries.

Strength training also improves cardiovascular fitness & general physical performance by building muscle endurance. The physiological demands of more strenuous cardiovascular activities, such as running, cycling, or swimming, can be better met by building stronger muscles.

Strength Training vs. Cardio for Weight Loss: A Comparison

Although they complement one another, cardiovascular exercise & strength training accomplish weight loss goals in distinct ways. In the short term, cardio works better for burning calories than other types of exercise because it raises heart rate & energy expenditure. Although regular steady-state cardio, such as jogging, can burn a lot of calories in a single session, HIIT increases calorie burn by a factor of two: during & after the workout.

But if you want to lose weight & burn fat permanently, strength training is a must. Although it may not result in a calorie deficit during exercise like cardio does, it does help build lean muscle mass, which raises resting metabolic rate. In the long run, losing fat may be easier if you gain muscle because your resting metabolic rate will be higher. When cutting calories is part of your weight loss or calorie restriction plan, strength training can help you maintain your muscle mass. The body may try to burn fat if it has enough muscle mass, but it may end up wasting muscle instead, which slows down metabolism & gives you that "skinny fat" appearance.

The best way to lose fat & get in the best shape of your life is to do a combination of cardiovascular exercise & strength training. While cardiovascular exercise can rapidly burn calories, strength training helps maintain or gain muscle, which in turn improves body composition & speeds up the metabolism.

Exploring the Health Benefits of Cardio & Strength Training

Incorporating both cardiovascular & strength training into your routine can help you live a healthier life. Cardiovascular exercises mainly help the cardiovascular system, which means they lower the risk of hypertension, heart disease, & stroke. Aerobic exercise improves cardiovascular health, which in turn increases oxygen uptake by working out the heart & lungs on a regular basis. Cardiovascular exercise also aids in making the body more insulin sensitive, which lowers the probability of developing type 2 diabetes.

When it comes to building & preserving muscle, increasing bone density, & enhancing joint health, strength training is paramount. Strength training aids mobility & functionality by increasing muscle mass & decreasing body fat. Injury prevention, especially for the elderly, depends on good posture, balance, & coordination, all of which it helps improve. Strength training also has positive effects on mental health, including increased self-confidence & less anxiety & depression.

Both kinds of physical activity have their advantages, but when done together, they have a multiplicative effect. Strength training can increase muscular endurance & handle more intense cardio, while cardiovascular exercise can improve the endurance needed for strength training. When combined, they form a well-rounded exercise program that takes a holistic approach to health & fitness by strengthening the muscles & the cardiovascular system.

The Importance of Regularity & Strength

Both the frequency & intensity of cardio & strength training affect their efficacy. HIIT & other forms of high-intensity interval training (HIIT) help you burn more calories in less time, increase metabolic flexibility, & boost your cardiovascular fitness quickly. Gains in muscular mass, strength, & endurance are possible outcomes of strength training when done at the right intensity. To maximize muscle growth & calorie expenditure during exercise & recovery, it is recommended to perform strength exercises with heavier weights or more complicated movements.

Cardio & strength training, like any other kind of exercise, work best when done regularly & with a steady progression. Consistent gains in strength & muscle mass can only be achieved through progressive overload, which entails progressively increasing the weight, resistance, or intensity of workouts. To improve cardiovascular health & fat loss, it is recommended to gradually increase the duration or intensity of cardiovascular exercises.

How About Both?

The answer to the question of whether strength training or cardio is superior is goal-specific. The best way to lose weight & burn fat is probably to do a mix of cardiovascular exercise & strength training. While cardiovascular exercise aids in generating the caloric deficit necessary for fat loss, strength training helps to increase muscle mass, which in turn boosts metabolism & promotes fat burning over the long term.

Due to its direct effects on cardiovascular function, cardiovascular exercise may take precedence for individuals whose goals include bettering lung & heart health, decreasing stress, & increasing stamina. However, strength training is crucial for those whose main objective is to gain muscle, improve strength, or delay the onset of age-related muscle atrophy. Additionally, it is essential for enhancing functional fitness & bone density, both of which are critical for preserving mobility in old age.

In summary

Choosing between cardiovascular exercise & strength training is not the answer to the question of which is more beneficial. In fact, for optimal health & fitness, it is best to incorporate both types of exercise into a combined program. This is because the two types of exercise complement one another & offer distinct but complementary advantages. Cardiovascular health, muscle mass, metabolism, & fat loss can all be enhanced with a well-rounded fitness program that incorporates strength training & cardiovascular exercise.

Whether your objective is to improve your general health, train for a particular event, or shed some pounds, a combination of cardiovascular exercise & strength training will help you get there faster & more efficiently.

Daily Movement for Sustainable Energy

The fast-paced nature of modern life frequently causes people to lead sedentary lives. Physical fitness often takes a back seat to other priorities, such as work, commute, & screen time. However, if you want to keep your energy levels, health, & vitality levels up over the long haul, you need to move every day. Incorporating movement into your daily routine can do more than just cramming in a few hours at the gym; it can rev up your metabolism, decrease fatigue, & improve your body's energy production & utilization efficiency. We optimize our mental outlook & the systems in our body that produce energy when we move regularly, which is an underappreciated but profoundly effective link between physical activity & energy. Exercising on a regular basis helps fight fatigue & keeps energy levels up all day long by improving circulation, boosting mitochondrial function, & enhancing the body's ability to use oxygen.

Maintaining a Regular Exercise Routine

The goal of sustainable energy is not merely to provide a short burst of energy to get things done; rather, it is to lay the groundwork for long-term physical, psychological, & emotional health. By getting your blood pumping on a daily basis, you can better supply your muscles & organs with oxygen & nutrients. Having a steady supply of oxygen is crucial for the proper functioning of the heart, lungs, & brain. Moving about helps the lymphatic system, which is involved in cleansing the body of toxins. Lymph fluid helps remove waste from the body, which supports cellular health & overall vitality. Movement promotes this flow.

Daily movement, even if just a little bit, can have a big impact on energy levels. Add as little as ten to fifteen minutes of physical activity to your daily schedule, & you'll feel more energized, less fatigued, & more productive, according to research. There will be noticeable benefits right away from a quick stroll, some light stretching, or some light yoga. Indulging in these activities can help alleviate stress & boost your mood by triggering the release of endorphins, which are the body's natural feel-good chemicals. We are less likely to experience mental or emotional fatigue & better able to conserve energy when stress levels are lower.

Energy Generation & Metabolism

Regular physical activity is essential for metabolic optimization, the process by which the body turns food into energy. The metabolic process is continuously at work in the body, metabolizing nutrients, producing energy, & controlling temperature & cell repair, among other functions. Walking, cycling, or other forms of low-intensity exercise, when practiced on a regular basis, help keep our metabolism running at full capacity. Rather than experiencing the energy slumps that many people feel after sitting for lengthy periods of time, this constant metabolic activity helps keep energy levels consistent throughout the day.

Getting some exercise every day also helps the mitochondria, the "powerhouses" of the cell that produce the energy our bodies need to operate. The molecule that powers cellular processes is produced by mitochondria & is known as adenosine triphosphate, or ATP. Fatigue & lethargy can result from impaired mitochondrial function, which can be caused by an inactive lifestyle. Physical activity increases energy production because it promotes mitochondrial biogenesis, or the creation of new mitochondria. Because this process improves energy efficiency, you won't need as many stimulants, like caffeine, to keep going strong.

Insulin sensitivity aids in the processing & storage of energy, & regular movement is an important component of this process. Metabolic function is improved when we move our bodies because it activates enzymes that aid in the burning of glucose for energy. You may feel more energized & have less weariness as a result of blood sugar imbalances if you do this.

The Importance of Adaptability & Power in Energy Control

Keep in mind that energy is about more than simply your heart rate. In order to keep energy levels sustainable, flexibility & strength are also crucial. By enhancing stability, stamina, & posture, muscular strength contributes to the body's overall function. Increasing our strength via weight-bearing exercises & resistance training not only makes us more physically capable, but it also makes us more physically resilient. Having strong muscles helps to stabilize the skeleton, eases pressure on the joints, & keeps you from suffering from the aches & pains that sap your energy.

On the flip side, being able to move freely helps alleviate stress & soreness. Everyday activities become more taxing when muscles are tense or constrained because they expend more energy when moving. A more relaxed state of mind &

more efficient use of energy can be yours after engaging in stretching & strengthening exercises like Pilates or yoga.

Emotional & Mental Vitality

Physical vitality is just one aspect of sustainable energy. The level of energy we experience on a daily basis is greatly influenced by our mental & emotional well-being. Exercising regularly releases feel-good neurochemicals like serotonin & dopamine, which enhance mental performance, concentration, & mood. These chemicals are crucial for controlling emotions, elevating mood, & sharpening focus. Reducing tension & anxiety through movement helps us keep our mental energy levels high. When you're under constant pressure, your body goes into "fight or flight" mode, which means it releases the stress hormone cortisol. This hormone can mess with your sleep schedule & sap your energy. Regular exercise helps to maintain a healthy cortisol level, which in turn promotes a relaxed, focused mindset that is conducive to increased energy & productivity.

Also, the quality of your sleep is significantly affected by how active you are. Our circadian rhythms, or the natural cycles of when we sleep & when we wake up, are better regulated when we move around on a regular basis. Because of this, you will be able to get the deeper, more rejuvenating sleep that your body & mind need. Getting enough sleep is essential for optimal bodily function; after all, our bodies are designed to recover through movement. Maintaining a regular exercise routine helps our bodies adjust to the demands of everyday life, which in turn increases our resilience & keeps us going for longer.

A Guide to Fitting Physical Activity Into Your Everyday Life

Finding the time to incorporate daily movement into hectic schedules is a challenge for many people. But you don't need to spend hours at the gym to get moving every day. To lead a more active lifestyle, it's important to incorporate small, consistent actions throughout the day. Here are some doable suggestions for fitting exercise into your daily routine:

To Get Your Blood Pumping & Your Body Moving First Thing in the Morning: Do some light stretching, yoga, or go for a quick walk to start your day off right. Your muscles & brain will get more oxygen, giving you more energy to start the day.

Get Up & Move About Every Half an Hour to an Hour If You Work at a Desk Job, Try to Stand Every Half an Hour to An Hour. Go for a short office stroll, stretch lightly, or do some basic bodyweight exercises like lunges or squats.

Instead of driving, try walking or riding a bike to work or when you need to run errands. If you must drive, park further away from your final destination so you can get more steps every day.

Doing things like gardening, playing with kids or pets, or even just cleaning up after yourself can be a terrific way to get some exercise & maintain your energy levels up all day long.

Wrap Up Your Day with Some Relaxation: Try some light yoga or stretching before bed to unwind, get a better night's sleep, & lessen nighttime restlessness. This will help you wake up feeling refreshed & ready to take on the day.

Sleep, Stress, & Hormones

The complex interplay of hormones, stress, & sleep is foundational to a robust metabolism & long-term energy stability. The state of one's physical, mental, & emotional health is affected by these three interconnected & mutually influential factors. Energy can be depleted, recovery slowed, & disease risk increased when disruptions in one area trigger imbalances in others. To optimize health, enhance metabolic function, & maintain long-term vitality, it is crucial to understand the interaction of hormones, stress, & sleep. In this chapter, we'll look at the physiological impacts of stress, the critical roles of sleep, & the ways hormones control these factors. We'll also look at some practical ways to balance these elements in our daily lives.

How Metabolism & Hormonal Balance Are Affected by Lack of Sleep

A good night's sleep is crucial to your health in general, but especially to the regulation of your metabolism & hormones. Repair, growth, & detoxification are three of the most important things that the body does while we sleep. Restorative sleep is essential for optimum metabolic function because it improves metabolic processes including fat metabolism, insulin sensitivity, & muscle repair. On the flip side, metabolic abnormalities such as impaired glucose metabolism, increased insulin resistance, & reduced fat oxidation are brought about by chronic sleep deprivation. Fatigue, excess weight, & metabolic disorders like type 2 diabetes & obesity are all brought on by these disruptions.

Insomnia can have a significant impact on many hormones, including insulin, which controls blood sugar levels. When you don't get enough shut-eye, your cells stop responding to insulin, which raises your blood sugar levels & causes your body to store more fat. This condition is known as insulin resistance. A good night's sleep is crucial for controlling blood sugar levels & maintaining a healthy weight because insulin resistance is a risk factor for metabolic syndrome & type 2 diabetes. Hormones that control hunger & fullness, ghrelin & leptin, are affected by sleep as well. Leptin tells the brain when you've eaten enough, while ghrelin, sometimes called the "hunger hormone," makes you want to eat more. Overeating & weight gain can occur as a result of increased hunger & cravings for high-calorie foods brought on by decreased leptin levels & increased ghrelin levels caused by sleep deprivation. The body's innate capacity to maintain a steady energy balance is thus undermined by the vicious cycle that results from insufficient sleep.

In addition to its critical role in metabolic processes, sleep is also involved in maintaining a healthy hormonal balance. Hormones like cortisol, growth hormone, & thyroid hormone are controlled by the body's circadian rhythm, which is a natural 24-hour cycle that controls sleep-wake patterns. When you don't get enough sleep, your circadian rhythm gets thrown off, which in turn affects your hormone levels & your overall well-being. For instance, deep sleep is the main time for the release of growth hormone, which plays an essential role in tissue repair, muscle growth, & fat metabolism. When you don't get enough sleep on a regular basis, your body produces less growth hormone, which hinders your ability to recover & gain muscle. In a similar vein, the main stress hormone in the body, cortisol, can have a negative effect on metabolism by encouraging fat storage, particularly in the abdominal region, when sleep is insufficient.

Hormones & Metabolism Affected by Stress

Although stress is always present, long-term stress can disrupt the body's metabolic rate & hormonal equilibrium. The body releases stress hormones like adrenaline & cortisol as part of its stress response, which is called the fight-or-flight reaction. Its purpose is to help us deal with immediate threats. In order to get the body ready for action, these hormones speed up the heart rate, raise the blood pressure, & give you more energy. Nevertheless, metabolic function can be negatively impacted when stress becomes chronic, as is often the case with job pressures, relationship problems, financial worries, & other persistent stressors.

The "stress hormone," or cortisol, is an essential component of the immune system's reaction to stress. Although cortisol plays an important role in maintaining normal blood sugar, metabolism, & immune response levels, it can cause a host of health issues when levels are consistently high. Abdominal fat storage, insulin resistance, hypertension, & immune suppression are all associated with prolonged cortisol elevation. In addition to worsening metabolic health, these alterations raise the probability of acquiring diseases like obesity, type 2 diabetes, & cardiovascular disease. Anxiety, sadness, & irritability are all symptoms of elevated cortisol levels, which add to the weariness one feels mentally & emotionally.

Adrenaline, also known as epiphanephrine, is released during times of acute stress & is another important hormone that is affected by stress. While adrenaline does improve performance in the short term, it can cause anxiety, insomnia, & hypertension if exposed to high doses for an extended period of time as a result of chronic stress. Burnout & energy depletion can set in when the body's capacity to adapt is overwhelmed by the continuous release of these stress hormones. Thyroid hormones are also affected by chronic stress. The thyroid is responsible for regulating metabolism, & stress can interfere with its release of hormones, which in turn disrupts thyroid function. This can worsen the low energy feeling by causing symptoms like lethargy, weight gain, & exhaustion.

A Trifecta of Sleep Deprivation, Stress, & Hormonal Discord

Hormones, stress, & sleep all have intricate & interdependent relationships. When you don't get enough sleep, your stress levels rise, which throws off your hormone balance. Lack of sleep, for instance, raises cortisol levels, which in turn can heighten anxiety & stress. This sets off a domino effect of stress & sleep deprivation, which in turn causes metabolic disturbance, impaired immune function, & chronic fatigue. Additionally, many people experience trouble sleeping due to stress, as elevated cortisol levels hinder the body's ability to relax & enter a restorative sleep state. Some people find it hard to fall asleep, stay asleep, or get into the deep, rejuvenating stages of sleep when they suffer from chronic stress. The cumulative effects of sleep deprivation & stress can be devastating to health, making it harder to recover, leaving you with less energy & putting you at greater risk of developing chronic diseases.

Sleep deprivation & chronic stress can disrupt hormone balance, which in turn impacts hunger & energy expenditure. Stress raises ghrelin levels & lowers leptin levels, which causes an increase in hunger & a desire for unhealthy food, as previously stated. Overeating, especially of fatty & sugary foods, can ensue, further interfering with metabolic health & leading to weight gain. Stress also triggers catabolism, the process by which the body releases energy for survival by breaking down muscles. Because muscle tissue burns more calories at rest than fat, this slows down your metabolism & hinders your ability to build & repair muscle. A vicious cycle of slowed metabolism, increased fat storage, & depleted energy levels can be created when stress & poor sleep are combined.

How to Get the Most Out of Your Sleep, Stress, & Hormones

Optimal metabolic function & energy levels are the result of well-managed sleep, stress, & hormones. Improving energy levels & hormone regulation can be as simple as making a nightly sleep routine a priority. This involves reducing exposure to blue light from screens in the hours preceding up to sleep, developing a soothing bedtime routine, & maintaining a regular sleep schedule. A proper functioning of hormones like growth hormone, insulin, & cortisol—all of which are vital for energy production & metabolism— depends on the body getting sufficient amounts of restorative sleep.

In order to keep your hormones in check & your energy levels up, stress management is essential. Reduce stress & cortisol production with techniques like progressive muscle relaxation, deep breathing exercises, & mindfulness meditation. Stress resilience & relaxation are both enhanced by regular physical activity like yoga or moderate-intensity exercise, which in turn supports hormonal balance. Furthermore, one can alleviate stress & enhance overall health by partaking in activities that bring them joy & relaxation, such as going for walks in nature, pursuing hobbies, or spending time with loved ones. Individuals can improve their metabolism, stabilize their hormones, & maintain energy levels all day long by establishing a routine that includes both stress reduction & rejuvenating sleep.

In summary

The complex interplay of hormones, stress, & sleep is a key factor in regulating our metabolism, energy levels, & general well-being. Hormonal imbalances brought on by insufficient sleep & persistent stress impair metabolism, cause weight gain, exhaustion, & burnout. On the flip side, if you want to get your hormones back in check, your metabolism in tip-top shape, & your energy production at its peak, focus on getting enough good sleep & managing your stress. Keeping sustainable energy & long-term vitality in check requires an understanding of & approach to the interrelated nature of hormones, stress, & sleep. Achieving optimal health & living a more energetic, vibrant life is possible when people implement strategies to enhance the quality of their sleep, manage their stress, & balance their hormones.

The Impact of Sleep on Metabolic Health

Numerous metabolic functions, including energy balance, insulin sensitivity, fat storage, & cellular repair, are impacted by sleep, making it an essential & complex regulator of metabolic health. The body carries out vital processes to keep homeostasis, control hormones, & promote cellular regeneration while we sleep, especially in the more advanced stages of REM. Chronic sleep loss or poor-quality sleep can cause several metabolic disturbances, such as impaired glucose metabolism, an increased risk of obesity, cardiovascular disease, & metabolic syndrome; thus, the significance of sleep for metabolic health cannot be emphasized enough. Disruptions to the body's internal circadian rhythm, which controls sleep-wake cycles, can have significant effects on metabolic function as a whole. Inadequate or irregular sleep, for example, can throw this rhythm off kilter. In addition to regulating hormones like insulin, cortisol, leptin, & ghrelin, sleep also influences fat metabolism, energy expenditure, & muscle repair, among other metabolic health-related processes. We can better grasp the significance of good sleep for avoiding metabolic diseases & preserving long-term health if we know how sleep affects metabolism.

Insulin is the hormone in charge of controlling blood sugar levels, & sleep is essential for its proper regulation. A steady blood sugar level is one benefit of getting a good night's rest, which also helps the body stay insulin sensitive. However, insulin resistance develops when the body's cells stop responding to insulin, which means the pancreas has to secrete more insulin to keep blood sugar levels normal. This happens when people don't get enough sleep or have trouble sleeping. Blood sugar levels, body fat percentage, & the likelihood of acquiring type 2 diabetes can all rise as a consequence of this cumulative stress on the pancreas. Sleep deprivation, even for as little as one night, can lower insulin sensitivity; however, prolonged sleep loss, over many weeks or months, can cause insulin resistance to become more pronounced, greatly raising the risk of metabolic diseases, according to studies. Additionally, glucose intolerance, in which the body has trouble absorbing & using glucose efficiently, increases the risk of fat storage & spikes in blood sugar, & is commonly associated with insufficient sleep. People who experience chronic sleep deprivation are more likely to develop diabetes & obesity due to these mechanisms, which affect the body's ability to metabolize food effectively.

The hormones ghrelin & leptin, which are associated with hunger, are also tightly regulated by sleep. The "hunger hormone," ghrelin, causes the brain to crave food, while the "stop eating" signal, leptin, tells the brain when it's full. Increased hunger & a desire for high-calorie, energy-dense foods are symptoms of sleep deprivation, which raises ghrelin levels & lowers leptin levels. Overeating & unhealthy food choices are encouraged by this imbalance, which leads to metabolic dysfunction & weight gain. In addition to adding to weight gain & making insulin resistance worse, sleep deprivation makes people crave sugary & fatty foods even more. Overeating, weight gain, & other disruptions to metabolic health can ensue from a lack of sleep, creating a vicious cycle. Body composition can undergo dramatic changes, such as an increase in fat storage & a decrease in lean muscle mass, when caloric intake is high & calorie processing efficiency is low. Because muscle tissue burns more calories when at rest than fat tissue, having a healthy amount of muscle mass is essential for a healthy metabolism. Because it alters body composition, sleep deprivation can affect metabolic rate & general health in the long run.

Fat metabolism & energy expenditure are two other important areas that sleep influences metabolism. The breakdown of stored fat for energy is one of the vital repair & restorative processes that the body undertakes while we sleep. Optimal fat metabolism occurs during the deeper stages of sleep, especially slow-wave sleep (SWS), when the body primarily uses energy from fat stores to repair & maintain cells. Maintaining a healthy body composition is made easier by this process, which promotes fat loss & supports metabolic health. On the other hand, if you have trouble falling or staying asleep, it might affect your metabolism & make you more likely to put on weight, especially around your middle. Heart disease, insulin resistance, & type 2 diabetes are all made more likely by visceral fat, which is a kind of abdominal fat. This makes it a major health concern. Sleep deprivation changes the body's fat-burning mechanisms, increasing the likelihood of fat storage rather than fat-burning, particularly in the abdominal region. Sleep deprivation has detrimental impacts on metabolic health, & this fat metabolism imbalance just makes things worse.

Sleep affects energy expenditure as well as glucose & fat metabolism. A lower resting metabolic rate (RMR) is associated with chronic sleep deprivation, according to the research. The RMR is the amount of energy used by the body while at rest to sustain essential functions like breathing, circulation, & cell production. It is easier to put on weight & more difficult to lose fat when the resting metabolic rate (RMR) is low because the body burns fewer calories all day long. Those whose metabolic processes are well-oiled from a good night's sleep, on the other hand, tend to expend more energy. Part of the reason for this is that the body can heal & restore its muscles while we sleep, & the amount of muscle mass plays a significant role in determining our metabolic rate. Muscles burn more calories even when they're not moving around, thanks to their higher metabolic rate compared to fat. Proper rest helps keep muscle mass, which means your metabolism will stay high & your energy expenditure will be more efficient.

Cortisol is a stress hormone, & sleep plays a significant role in its hormonal regulation. Inflammation, glucose metabolism, & fat storage are all impacted by the stress hormone cortisol. On the other hand, increased cortisol levels, which occur when sleep is disturbed, can cause fat storage, especially in the abdominal area. The body's ability to process glucose efficiently can be hindered by chronic elevation of cortisol caused by inadequate sleep, which in turn impairs insulin sensitivity. Exacerbating weight gain & metabolic dysfunction, elevated cortisol levels are linked to increased hunger & cravings for unhealthy foods. The secretion of growth hormone—vital for repairing damaged tissues, building muscle, & metabolizing fat—can also be disrupted by elevated cortisol levels. Inadequate sleep reduces levels of growth hormone, which hinders the body's capacity to repair tissues, build muscle, & regulate fat metabolism. This crucial hormone is mainly released during deep sleep.

In addition, the internal clock of the body known as circadian rhythms controls the release of hormones, metabolic rates, & the duration & quality of sleep. Being consistent with your sleep-wake cycles is important because your circadian rhythms affect when your body uses energy, stores fat, & how sensitive insulin is. Impairments in glucose metabolism, insulin resistance, & increased fat storage have been linked to circadian misalignment, which can be caused by shift work, jet lag, or irregular sleep schedules, among other disruptions to circadian rhythms. Specifically, night shift workers are more likely to suffer from metabolic syndrome, obesity, & type 2 diabetes due to their often misaligned circadian rhythms. You can regulate your circadian rhythms & improve your metabolic health by sticking to a regular sleep schedule & adjusting your sleep to coincide with the natural light-dark cycle.

Noteworthy as well is the correlation between a good night's sleep & cardiometabolic wellness. Insomnia is associated with an increased risk of cardiovascular disease & other metabolic abnormalities, including insulin resistance, hypertension, & dyslipidemia. Conditions like hypertension, atherosclerosis, & stroke—all of which are associated with metabolic dysfunction—are more likely to develop in people who suffer from chronic sleep deprivation. Hormonal regulation, especially the effects of growth hormone, insulin, & cortisol on the cardiovascular system, primarily mediates the relationship between sleep & cardiovascular health. As an example, the heart & blood vessels are already under a lot of stress from things like elevated blood pressure, increased heart rate, & vasoconstriction (the narrowing of blood vessels) caused by high cortisol levels from not getting enough sleep.

Finally, getting enough sleep is crucial for keeping your metabolism in tip-top shape. Metabolic function & long-term health are impacted by its crucial role in controlling glucose metabolism, fat storage, energy expenditure, & hormonal balance. Insulin resistance, excess body fat, & an increased risk of metabolic disorders like type 2 diabetes, cardiovascular disease, & metabolic syndrome are just a few of the metabolic disturbances that can result from chronic sleep loss, poor-quality sleep, or irregular sleep patterns. To support metabolic health & lower the risk of developing chronic health problems, it is essential to prioritize quality sleep, maintain consistent sleep schedules, & address sleep disturbances. Now that we know how sleep affects metabolism, we can take measures to guarantee that we get the rejuvenating sleep that our metabolisms need to work at their best & keep us healthy for the long haul.

Managing Stress for Better Energy

To keep your energy levels & metabolism in tip-top shape, stress management is a must. Disruption of numerous physiological systems by chronic stress can result in exhaustion, impaired metabolic function, & the onset of chronic diseases. We can safeguard our energy stores, speed up our metabolism, & promote our physical & mental well-being by mastering the art of stress management. The sympathetic nervous system is activated & stress hormones like adrenaline & cortisol are released, which have an impact on the body. Although temporary stress aids in responding to urgent dangers, long-term stress causes these hormones to remain elevated, which has negative impacts on energy levels & metabolism.

An important mechanism by which stress influences metabolism is via its influence on cortisol, commonly known as the "stress hormone." A number of detrimental metabolic effects can occur when cortisol levels stay elevated due to chronic stress. A hormone called cortisol raises blood sugar levels by causing the liver to release glucose into the bloodstream. This process can eventually cause insulin resistance. Insulin plays a crucial role in controlling blood sugar & fat storage, but when the body develops insulin resistance, it becomes less responsive to the hormone. This causes problems with glucose metabolism & may encourage fat storage, especially around the middle. Hormones like ghrelin & leptin are involved in controlling hunger, & elevated cortisol levels can interfere with their function. Leptin indicates fullness, while ghrelin promotes hunger. The hunger hormone ghrelin can rise in response to stress, leading to increased calorie, sugar, & fat consumption as well as the desire for so-called "comfort foods." A higher risk of metabolic diseases like type 2 diabetes, poor energy regulation, & weight gain can ensue from this vicious cycle of overeating & impaired glucose metabolism.

The autonomic nervous system is influenced by stress as well. This system controls involuntary functions like digestion, energy production, & heart rate. The sympathetic nervous system, which initiates the "fight or flight" reaction, can remain constantly activated in people who experience chronic stress. Although this comes in handy in an emergency, it can drain your energy reserves & leave you feeling mentally & physically tired if it's activated for too long. Feelings of exhaustion are exacerbated by nutrient depletion, which occurs when the body's demand for nutrients is increased due to the constant demand for energy during stressful periods. When the stress response is kept on for too long, it can wear down the adrenal glands, which are responsible for producing hormones like cortisol, to the point where they no longer function as effectively. This condition is known as adrenal fatigue. Difficulty focusing, disturbed sleep patterns, & persistent tiredness are all possible outcomes.

To avoid these detrimental impacts on energy & metabolism, it is essential to manage stress effectively. Research has demonstrated that engaging in mindfulness practices such as yoga, deep breathing, & meditation can alleviate stress & lower cortisol levels in the body. By making these routines a part of your life, you can train your parasympathetic nervous system to take over digestion, repair, & relaxation, rather than the fight-or-flight response. Practicing mindfulness, even for short intervals throughout the day, can have a positive effect on energy levels & the autonomic nervous system. Consistent physical exercise, along with mindfulness practices, can be an effective means of alleviating stress. Exercise improves energy management in multiple ways: by regulating cortisol levels, by promoting the release of endorphins (the body's natural mood enhancers), & by improving sleep. However, you should not overdo it when it comes to exercise; doing too much too soon can raise cortisol levels & cause overtraining, so make sure to include both active & rest periods in your schedule.

Another important part of stress management & energy conservation is getting enough sleep. The physiological & psychological effects of stress can be alleviated through the restorative process that occurs during sleep. As the body enters a restorative state during deep sleep, cortisol levels inevitably fall. Conversely, stress can worsen when you don't get enough sleep because it increases cortisol production, hinders cognitive function, & lowers your body's stress tolerance. To improve the quality of your sleep & lessen the weariness that comes from stress, it's important to establish a regular sleep schedule, learn relaxation techniques before bed, & make your bedroom a relaxing place to sleep.

A healthy diet is also important for regulating stress & keeping energy levels stable. The body's stress tolerance & energy regulation mechanisms are both bolstered by nutrient-dense meals, especially those abundant in antioxidants, vitamins, & minerals. For optimal neurological health & stress response regulation, eat plenty of B-vitamin-rich foods like legumes, leafy greens, & whole grains. Consuming magnesium-rich foods, such as nuts, seeds, & dark chocolate, can help lower cortisol levels & induce a calming effect on the body. Fatty fish, flaxseeds, & walnuts are good sources of omega-3 fatty acids, which have anti-inflammatory characteristics & can help mitigate stress's harmful effects on the body. Because they cause cortisol spikes & subsequent energy crashes, sugar & caffeine should also be avoided to the extreme. Alternatively, you can support your body's stress response & have sustained energy by concentrating on balanced meals that include lean proteins, complex carbs, & healthy fats.

Another important factor in stress management is having strong relationships & social support. When people have people they can lean on in times of need, whether it be friends, family, or coworkers, it can alleviate emotional pain, lessen feelings of loneliness, & improve resilience. Restoring energy levels & improving metabolic health are two benefits of social interaction that are accompanied by the release of the stress-relieving & relaxation-promoting hormone oxytocin. You can change your body's reaction to stress by getting help when you need it, whether that's through therapy or just talking to someone you trust.

A more balanced stress response & improved energy regulation can be achieved by incorporating these strategies into daily life. To maintain one's physical & mental health, it is essential to learn to cope with stress, which is an unavoidable aspect of living. Protecting our energy reserves, improving our metabolism, & enhancing our overall health can be accomplished by prioritizing stress-reduction practices like regular exercise, mindful relaxation, good sleep hygiene, & nutritious food.

All things considered, stress significantly alters metabolic rate & energy reserves. Our metabolism, fat storage, glucose regulation, & general health can all benefit from better stress management, which in turn mitigates the negative effects of cortisol & other stress hormones. Mindfulness, exercise, healthy eating, & sufficient sleep are some of the most important techniques for stress management & energy preservation. In a world where stress is ever-present, incorporating these practices into our daily routine can assist in maintaining our health, energy, & resilience.

Hormonal Balance & Metabolism

The metabolic process—the body's way of turning food into energy & controlling the storage & utilization of nutrients—is heavily influenced by hormones. The thyroid, adrenal glands, pancreas, & reproductive organs are among the glands that produce these biochemical messengers, which aid in the regulation of multiple metabolic processes. For optimum energy levels, weight control, & general health, a metabolic system that is well-balanced is crucial. Tiredness, gaining weight, trouble losing weight, or metabolic disorders like hypothyroidism or diabetes can be symptoms of a hormonal imbalance that throws the body's metabolism out of whack.

1. Hormones Produced by the Thyroid & Their Role in Metabolism: Neck-based thyroid gland hormones like thyroxine (T4) & triiodothyronine (T3) play an essential role in controlling metabolic rate. These hormones regulate the body's sensitivity to other hormones, speed up or slow down energy utilization, & affect protein synthesis. Symptoms of hyperthyroidism, or an overactive thyroid, include a rapid metabolism, rapid heart rate, anxiety, & decreased body fat. In contrast, hypothyroidism (an underactive thyroid) causes a slowed metabolism, which in turn causes extra weight to accumulate, extreme weariness, & trouble focusing. Inadequate nutrition, stress, & autoimmune diseases can all interfere with thyroid hormone production, which in turn

can disrupt metabolic function, which is crucial for maintaining a balanced metabolic rate.

2. The Metabolism of Insulin & Glucose: The pancreatic hormone insulin is essential for maintaining normal blood sugar levels & for storing energy. Insulin facilitates the absorption of glucose (sugar) from the bloodstream after food consumption, allowing cells to either use it for energy or store it for later use. Stable blood sugar levels, maintained by an efficient insulin system, supply a steady stream of energy all day long. It becomes difficult for the body to maintain normal blood sugar levels when insulin production is inadequate or when cells develop a resistance to insulin. Fatigue, weight gain, & type 2 diabetes are possible outcomes. Factors such as an unhealthy diet, insufficient physical activity, & chronic stress can lead to insulin resistance, which in turn hinders metabolic function.

3. The adrenal glands secrete cortisol, the principal hormone that the body uses to respond to stress. In times of stress, it increases glucose production & mobilizes stored fats for fuel, two crucial functions in energy regulation. Prolonged elevation of cortisol levels can be caused by chronic stress, in contrast to the short-term increases that are helpful in responding to acute stress. Prompting insulin resistance & increasing fat storage (especially in the abdominal region), this chronic stress can throw metabolism for a loop. In addition to exacerbating metabolic problems, elevated cortisol levels can disrupt thyroid function. Keeping cortisol levels under control & metabolic balance intact requires stress management strategies such as relaxation techniques, exercise, & adequate sleep.

Leptin & ghrelin, the hormones that control hunger:

Fat storage, energy expenditure, & the regulation of hunger & satiety are all affected by the hormones leptin & ghrelin. Fat cells secrete leptin, commonly known as the "satiety hormone," which tells the brain that there is an adequate supply of energy & causes hunger to decrease. On the other hand, the stomach secretes ghrelin, also called the "hunger hormone," which increases hunger & makes the body want to eat. Overeating, excess weight gain, & metabolic dysregulation can result from an imbalance in these two hormones. Chronic stress, sleep deprivation, & obesity can reduce leptin sensitivity, making it harder for the body to signal satiety effectively, leading to overeating & weight gain.

5. Estrogen & Metabolism: Estrogen, the primary female sex hormone, also plays a significant role in metabolism. It influences how the body stores fat, regulates energy expenditure, & manages glucose metabolism. During perimenopause & menopause, estrogen levels naturally decline, which can lead to an increase in abdominal fat, a decrease in muscle mass, & changes in insulin sensitivity. These changes may make weight management & maintaining energy levels more challenging. Low estrogen levels also slow the metabolism & make it harder for the body to burn fat, which can lead to weight gain. Maintaining a balanced hormonal environment through diet, exercise, & stress management can help support estrogen levels & improve metabolic function during this life stage.

6. Testosterone & Metabolism: Testosterone, primarily known as a male sex hormone, also plays a vital role in metabolism for both men & women. It helps regulate muscle mass, fat distribution, & bone density, all of which are closely linked to metabolic health. Testosterone increases the body's ability to burn fat & build muscle, both of which are essential

for maintaining a healthy metabolism. Low testosterone levels, which occur naturally in both sexes as we get older, are associated with a loss of muscular mass, gain of fat, & a slowing of the metabolic rate. For a balanced metabolism, it's important to keep testosterone levels in a healthy range through exercise (especially strength training), good nutrition, & getting enough sleep.

7. Growth Hormone & Repair: The pituitary gland secretes growth hormone (GH), which aids in cell proliferation, tissue regeneration, & the development of muscles. Stimulating the breakdown of fat stores for energy, it plays a crucial role in fat metabolism. Loss of growth hormone with age is a known cause of aging-related changes in body composition, including less muscle mass, more fat, & a slower metabolism. To promote healthy metabolic function & increase production of natural growth hormone, it is essential to get enough sleep, train with resistance, & eat well.

8. Maintaining Hormonal Balance for Metabolic Health: Since hormones are so important for metabolism, it stands to reason that maintaining hormonal balance is key to regulating energy effectively, burning fat, & having a healthy metabolism in general. Hormonal balance can be disturbed by a number of things, such as an unhealthy diet, stress, lack of physical activity, inadequate sleep, & environmental pollutants. Hormonal balance & metabolic health can be optimized by adopting a lifestyle that supports healthy hormone production & regulation. This includes eating nutrient-dense foods, being physically active on a regular basis, managing stress, & making sleep a priority.

The role of hormones in controlling metabolic rate & maintaining homeostasis of energy is, thus, crucial. Weight gain, exhaustion, & other metabolic disorders can result from hormonal imbalances including thyroid hormones, insulin, cortisol, leptin, ghrelin, estrogen, testosterone, & growth hormone. Supporting metabolic function & promoting sustained energy levels requires achieving & maintaining hormonal balance through lifestyle practices like a healthy diet, regular exercise, stress management, & proper sleep. Gaining insight into the relationship between hormones & metabolism will empower you to take charge of your health & reach your metabolic potential.

Environmental & Lifestyle Factors

The rate at which our bodies turn food into energy, store fat, & regulate metabolic health is influenced by a multitude of environmental & lifestyle factors, in addition to genetics & internal biological processes. If we are aware of the ways in which these environmental factors can help or hurt metabolic function, we can make decisions that are best for our metabolic health. A person's ability to keep their metabolic rate healthy is influenced by a number of factors. These include their food, level of physical activity, amount of sleep they get, stress levels, environmental pollutants, & social determinants such as their socioeconomic status & access to healthcare.

1. Eating Habits & the Food System

An individual's metabolic health is critically affected by the food environment, which in turn determines the quality of the diet. A well-functioning metabolism is supported by a nutrient-dense diet that includes whole foods like fruits, vegetables, lean meats, healthy fats, & whole grains, as opposed to processed & refined foods that are rich in added sugars, trans fats, & sodium. In particular, insulin spikes caused by eating too much sugar encourage fat storage & may eventually cause insulin resistance. Similarly, a spike in blood sugar from eating too many refined carbs can cause an overproduction of insulin, which in turn can cause energy crashes & encourage fat storage. Conversely, a healthy metabolism is supported by a diet rich in lean proteins, fiber-rich veggies, & healthy fats such as those found in avocados, nuts, & olive oil. These foods all work together to stabilise blood sugar levels, enhance fat-burning processes, & support hormonal balance.

The rhythm & sequence of meals also have an effect on metabolic rate. For instance, research has demonstrated that intermittent fasting—a practice in which people alternate between eating & not eating—can enhance fat oxidation, insulin sensitivity, & autophagy, the body's mechanism for removing damaged cells. Additionally, it is important to consider the variety & quality of food available to us. Poor eating habits, increased obesity rates, & impaired metabolic function are associated with places that do not have easy access to fresh, nutritious food. These places are called food deserts. To improve metabolic health for all, these environmental inequalities highlight the necessity for legislative changes that expand access to nutritious foods.

2. Moving About & Avoiding Inactivity

One of the most powerful metabolic enhancers is regular physical activity, which improves nutrient utilisation, fat burning, & muscle mass gain. To raise the metabolic rate, one can engage in aerobic exercise like jogging, swimming, or cycling, as well as strength training like lifting weights or resistance exercises. For example, aerobic exercise has many health benefits, including better heart health, better mitochondrial function, & increased fat oxidation both during exercise & at rest. On the flip side, one's resting metabolic rate (RMR)—the quantity of energy used by the body while at rest—is elevated after strength training due to the increased muscle mass.

Alternatively, sitting for long periods of time or engaging in other forms of inactivity can drastically reduce metabolic function, leading to increased risk of obesity, type 2 diabetes, insulin resistance, & cardiovascular disease. One of the leading causes of poor metabolic health in modern society is the rise of sedentary lifestyles, which are caused by desk jobs, increased screen time, & technological advancements that reduce physical movement. Incorporating more movement into your daily routine, standing desks, or taking short walks can help combat the negative effects of a sedentary lifestyle & enhance metabolic function.

3. Metabolic Sleep

Maintaining metabolic health relies on sleep, which is frequently disregarded despite its critical importance. The body's capacity to regulate hormones that control hunger & metabolism can be disrupted by poor sleep quality, which can be caused by sleep disorders like sleep apnoea or by lifestyle factors like using screens too close to bedtime or having irregular sleep schedules. The hormones leptin & ghrelin are responsible for signalling fullness & hunger, respectively; when people don't get enough sleep, the balance of these hormones is upset, which can lead to weight gain, increased hunger, & cravings for high-calorie foods. In addition to slowing metabolic processes, high levels of the stress hormone cortisol, which can be caused by chronic sleep deprivation, encourage fat storage & insulin resistance.

A healthy metabolism relies on repairing & regenerating cells & tissues, both of which are essential functions of sleep. A lack of sleep is associated with metabolic syndrome & other long-term health problems including impaired glucose tolerance, increased inflammation, & decreased insulin sensitivity. Making sleep a top priority & practicing good sleep hygiene (e.g., sticking to a regular sleep schedule, developing a relaxing bedtime routine, & making sure your bedroom is cool & dark) can have positive effects on hormone regulation, energy levels, & metabolism.

4. Cortisol & Stress

A person's metabolic rate can also be affected by chronic stress. Cortisol is the principal stress hormone released by the body when it undergoes sympathetic nervous system activation in response to stress. Although cortisol plays a crucial role in alleviating temporary stress, it can cause metabolic disruptions when levels of chronic stress remain consistently high. Elevated cortisol levels are associated with an increase in food cravings, especially for calorie-heavy foods, & with the development of abdominal fat. In addition to increasing fat storage & exhaustion, cortisol has a deleterious effect on insulin sensitivity, making it more difficult for the body to control blood sugar levels.

A decrease in cortisol levels, an improvement in metabolic function, & support for general well-being can result from stress management strategies such as meditation, deep breathing, & frequent exercise. Support from friends & family, a healthy work-life balance, & easy access to mental health services are all examples of environmental & social variables that impact stress resilience.

5. Pollutants in the Environment

The effects of environmental pollutants on metabolism & general health have been the subject of increasing public attention in recent years. Research has demonstrated that endocrine-disrupting chemicals (EDCs) like bisphenol A (BPA), phthalates, & specific pesticides can disrupt metabolic processes by interfering with hormone production & function. These chemicals can imitate or inhibit the actions of natural hormones like oestrogen, testosterone, & thyroid hormones; they are ubiquitous in plastics, food packaging, & common household things. Impaired metabolic health can result from disruptions in these hormones, which in turn can cause weight gain, insulin resistance, & thyroid dysfunction.

Chronic inflammation, which environmental pollutants exacerbate, can throw off metabolism even more, leading to health problems like diabetes, obesity, & cardiovascular disease. Choosing BPA-free products, eating organic foods, & using natural cleaning products can help reduce exposure to environmental toxins, which can help mitigate their effects on metabolism & promote long-term health.

6. Factors Influencing Social Determinants & Resource Access

Lastly, metabolic health can be impacted by socioeconomic determinants including education level, income, healthcare access, & community resources. Inadequate access to healthcare, safe places to exercise, & nutritious food is a common problem among people from lower socioeconomic backgrounds, & it can have a negative effect on metabolism. Poor food choices, increased obesity rates, & impaired metabolic function can be observed in areas where fresh, affordable food is scarce, known as a food desert. Diabetes & hypothyroidism, for example, can go untreated due to a lack of access to healthcare, leading to additional metabolic dysfunction.

Improving metabolic health & making sure everyone has a chance to thrive requires addressing these social disparities through community-based interventions & changes to policies.

The Role of Toxins & Pollutants

It is becoming more & more apparent that environmental pollutants & toxins significantly impair metabolic health. Pollutants in the air, water, food, & soil can cause long-term health problems by interfering with the body's metabolic processes & introducing hazardous substances like heavy metals & chemicals. Hormonal disruption, increased inflammation, insulin resistance, & changes in fat storage are just a few of the many ways these pollutants impact metabolism. Toxins are becoming more ubiquitous in our daily lives & the world around us, so it's important to know how they affect metabolism so we can protect our health in the long run.

First, hormonal imbalance & endocrine-disrupting chemicals (EDCs)

Concerningly, environmental pollutants can interfere with the endocrine system, which is responsible for controlling metabolism & other critical bodily functions through its intricate network of glands & hormones. In order to disrupt metabolic function, endocrine-disrupting chemicals (EDCs) can imitate or interfere with the body's natural hormones. Packaging for food & personal care items, as well as industrial chemicals, frequently contain these substances.

Among the most common EDCs are pesticides, dioxins, phthalates, PCBs, & bisphenol A (BPA). Because of their ubiquitous presence in nature, they pose a threat to human health when ingested, come into touch with skin, or inhaled.

The regulation of fat storage, muscle mass, energy expenditure, & glucose metabolism can be disrupted when EDCs imitate or inhibit the actions of hormones like thyroid, oestrogen, & testosterone. For example, bisphenol A (BPA), which is present in many food & drink containers, can impair insulin action, which in turn increases the likelihood of developing insulin resistance & type 2 diabetes. Additionally, BPA & related compounds can promote abdominal obesity, which is associated with metabolic diseases, & hence can affect fat accumulation.

Second, Insulin Resistance & Toxins

A major metabolic impact of environmental pollutants is the development of insulin resistance, a state in which cells in the body lose some of their sensitivity to the hormone responsible for controlling blood sugar levels. Metabolic disorders including metabolic syndrome, obesity, & type 2 diabetes all share insulin resistance as a defining characteristic. Toxins from chemicals & pollutants in particular can disrupt insulin signalling pathways, which in turn causes problems with glucose metabolism & an increase in fat storage.

Insulin resistance is more likely to occur in people who are exposed to certain environmental pollutants, such as EDCs, heavy metals, & air pollutants. For instance, research has demonstrated that adipose tissue (fat cells) function can be altered by exposure to persistent organic pollutants (POPs), a class of harmful chemicals that build up in the environment

& food chain. This, in turn, can lead to insulin resistance. An increase in fat deposition & a decrease in insulin sensitivity have been associated with PCBs, a kind of POP. Similarly, impaired glucose metabolism, an increased risk of obesity & diabetes, & mercury exposure—often through contaminated fish—have been linked.

3. Metabolic Dysfunctionand/or Inflammation

In addition to their effects on metabolism, environmental pollutants can trigger chronic inflammation. While inflammation is an immune system reaction to harm, it can lead to metabolic dysfunction if it lasts too long. Obesity, insulin resistance, atherosclerosis, & type 2 diabetes are metabolic diseases characterised by low-grade chronic inflammation.

Air pollution, pesticides, & industrial chemicals are just a few examples of the many environmental pollutants that have been proven to cause inflammatory reactions in living organisms. These inflammatory processes change the function of important metabolic organs like the liver & muscles, promote fat storage, & interfere with insulin signalling. Chronic inflammation, brought on by air pollution, especially PM2.5, can worsen insulin resistance & throw off fat metabolism. Likewise, research has demonstrated that heavy metal exposure, including lead & cadmium, raises inflammatory marker levels, which in turn contributes to metabolic dysfunction.

4. Body Fat Percentage & Obesity

Toxins in the environment also play a major role in how fat is distributed & how obesity develops. Metabolic illness is closely linked to abdominal obesity, which is exacerbated by many pollutants, particularly EDCs. The metabolic activity, hormones, & inflammatory molecules released by visceral fat (fat stored around the organs) make it a particularly dangerous kind of fat. Evidence suggests that phthalates, dioxins, & bisphenol A (BPA) impede the body's natural fat storage regulation mechanisms, leading to increased belly fat. Cardiovascular disease, type 2 diabetes, & other metabolic diseases may become more likely as a result of this.

According to some research, EDCs have a dual effect: they enhance fat storage & change the way fat cells work, either making them less efficient at burning fat or more likely to store it. These pollutants have the ability to impact fat cell development during early life, which could have long-term effects on metabolic health & body composition as an adult. Some chemicals can change a developing baby's metabolism during pregnancy, increasing the likelihood that the child will be overweight or suffer from a metabolic disorder later in life.

5. Environmental Harm & Mitochondrial Impairment

The "powerhouses" of the cell, the mitochondria, are in charge of producing ATP, the cellular energy currency. Because it controls the body's capacity to burn fat, use glucose, & generate energy, mitochondrial function is crucial for efficient metabolism. Research has demonstrated that heavy metals, pesticides, solvents, & other environmental pollutants can hinder mitochondrial function, resulting in energy inefficiency & disruptions to metabolic processes.

For instance, research has connected lead exposure to mitochondrial dysfunction, which in turn can increase fat storage & decrease energy production efficiency.

Organochlorine pesticides have similar detrimental effects on mitochondrial function, which in turn cause inflammation, impaired fat metabolism, & increased oxidative stress.

Section 6: The Liver & Detoxification

Metabolic processes, such as glucose storage & fat-to-energy conversion, are regulated by the liver, which also plays an important role in detoxifying toxic substances. But the liver can only detoxify so much before it gets fatty liver disease & other metabolic malfunctions from being exposed to environmental pollutants for too long. Toxins like alcohol, heavy metals, & processed food chemicals can irritate & stress the liver, which in turn hinders its capacity to control glucose & lipid metabolism.

Fat buildup in the liver without alcohol consumption is known as non-alcoholic fatty liver disease (NAFLD), & metabolic dysfunction is closely associated with this condition. Insulin resistance & fat storage are worsened by toxins that cause non-alcoholic fatty liver disease (NAFLD), which include chemicals found in processed foods & air pollution. To keep metabolic health, it is essential to support liver health through detoxification, a healthy diet, & limiting exposure to environmental pollutants.

7. Methods for Prevention & Minimising Risk

Toxins & pollutants have a worrying effect on the environment, but there are ways people can lessen their exposure & lessen the impact on their metabolism. You can lessen your exposure to dangerous chemicals by eating organic foods, cutting back on plastic use, & staying away from products that contain bisphenol A. Improving indoor air quality & reducing toxic exposure can be achieved with the help of air purifiers & cleaning products derived from plants. Oxidative stress from pollutants can be mitigated by eating more antioxidant-rich foods, like berries, leafy greens, & cruciferous vegetables.

When dealing with environmental pollutants, regular exercise is a potent tool for improving metabolic health. By increasing the body's natural detoxification processes, decreasing inflammation, & enhancing insulin sensitivity, exercise mitigates the metabolic impacts of pollutants. By regulating hormones & reducing inflammation, stress management techniques & getting enough sleep both help the body deal with environmental pollutants.

Digital Detox: Reducing Screen Time for Energy

The pervasiveness of screens in today's always-on, always-connected world has revolutionised the way we go about our everyday lives. Our mental & physical health are suffering as a result of the growing amount of time spent in front of screens, be they smartphones, laptops, tablets, or televisions. Excessive use of technology has been associated to numerous negative health outcomes, such as exhaustion, disturbed sleep, elevated stress levels, & metabolic disturbances, despite the fact that it has brought numerous conveniences. Recognising the importance of taking breaks & embracing a digital detox to restore energy & improve overall metabolic health has become crucial as our digital lives become more intertwined with our real-world activities.

1. The Metabolic Effects of Screen Addiction

Loss of physical activity is one of the first & most obvious consequences of spending too much time in front of screens. A sedentary lifestyle is exacerbated by the fact that many people spend long periods of time sitting, frequently in front of screens. Insulin resistance, obesity, cardiovascular disease, & other metabolic disorders are all increased by leading an inactive lifestyle. The capacity of the body to metabolise glucose & fat is negatively impacted by sitting for long periods of time, as is shown in numerous studies. Slower metabolism, more fat storage, & elevated blood sugar levels are all symptoms of metabolic dysfunction that can result from this.

Disrupting the body's natural rhythms adds insult to injury when combined with the lack of movement caused by screen time. An active metabolism is essential for good health because it increases energy expenditure & the growth of muscle. However, this process is slowed down & metabolic health can be negatively affected in the long run by sitting for lengthy periods of time, particularly when movement is minimal. Thus, in order to keep a healthy metabolism, it is essential to reduce screen time & increase physical activity throughout the day.

2. The Effects of Screen Time on Sleep

Overexposure to screens also has a major effect on sleep quality, which in turn slows metabolism. In particular, exposure to blue light from screens in the hours leading up to bedtime prevents the body from making the sleep-inducing hormone melatonin. The production of melatonin, a hormone that tells the body it's time to relax & get ready for sleep, is crucial. But nighttime blue light exposure can postpone melatonin release, which makes falling asleep & staying asleep more difficult & less restful.

Sleep deprivation has a direct & negative effect on metabolic health. Sleep deprivation is associated with insulin resistance, high cortisol levels, & impaired regulation of hunger hormones such as leptin & ghrelin, according to research. Overeating, increased desire for high-calorie foods, & excess weight gain are all possible outcomes of these changes. Inadequate sleep also interferes with the body's natural capacity to repair tissues, control energy balance, & keep metabolic processes in good shape. In order to promote a healthier metabolism & get a better night's sleep, it's recommended to avoid using electronic devices for at least an hour before bed.

3. Reducing Stress through Digital Means

Overexposure to screens is associated with negative effects on mental & emotional health as well as physical health. An increase in cortisol levels, a stress hormone with systemic effects, can be caused by being "always on" & constantly checking notifications, scrolling through social media, & other screens. Elevated cortisol levels, especially in the abdominal region, can lead to insulin resistance, hormonal imbalance, & the development of visceral fat.

Reducing cortisol levels & increasing relaxation can be achieved through regular device breaks, such as a digital detox. People can support metabolic health & reduce the risk of stress-induced metabolic disorders by engaging in stress-reducing activities like mindful breathing, yoga, or spending time in nature during these detox periods. Better control of cortisol levels & protection of metabolic function can be achieved through less screen time & the promotion of a peaceful, stress-free environment.

4. Enhancing Concentration & Vitality With the Help of a Digital Fast

Taking a break from technology can boost concentration & clarity of thought, which in turn can increase energy & output. It can be challenging to focus on critical tasks or make significant advancements in our personal & professional lives when we are continually inundated with notifications, emails, & social media updates. Continuously shifting between tasks, also known as multitasking or task-switching, decreases our mental efficiency & amplifies feelings of mental exhaustion, leaving us feeling depleted & lacking in energy.

Our brains need time to recharge, so we should limit our screen usage & instead focus on one thing at a time or do things that encourage mindfulness, like reading, writing, or going for walks in nature. Improved mental clarity, increased stamina, & enhanced cognitive function are all benefits of this. Improved mood, increased vitality, & increased productivity are all possible outcomes.

5. Regulating Screen Time in a Healthy Way

While it may not be practical or feasible to totally cut out screen time, there are a number of ways to lessen screen time that still promote metabolic health & general wellness. In order to establish more beneficial routines involving screen time, here are some suggestions:

Limit Your Screen Time: You can use apps or your phone's settings to keep tabs on how much time you spend staring at your screen. To avoid becoming addicted & to promote a more balanced day, try setting a time limit for yourself each day for things like social media & television.

For better sleep, avoid using electronic devices for at least an hour before turning in. Instead, try reading, meditating, or keeping a journal to help your body relax & wind down.

If you find yourself spending long periods of time in front of a screen, whether it's a computer, phone, or tablet, schedule brief breaks every 30 to 60 minutes. A better circulation & less metabolic impact from sitting for long periods can be achieved by getting up & moving about, stretching, or doing some exercise.

Exercising: Make the most of your time away from screens by engaging in physical activity. Incorporating regular physical activity into your routine, be it a walk, workout, or yoga, can counteract the negative impacts of inactivity & enhance energy levels.

Turn off or put your phone in another room if you don't want to be interrupted while you eat. The result is enhanced digestion & more mindful eating, both of which have a favourable effect on metabolism.

Make Some Rooms in Your House Off-Limits Electronic Devices: Set aside specific rooms in your house, like the bedroom or the dining room, to promote rest & in-person communication free of screen time.

6. Technology Use with Caution

Even though it's good to spend less time in front of screens, technology isn't bad in & of itself. The key is in our application. To make sure that screens enrich our lives instead of diminishing them, it's important to use technology mindfully. Some ways to accomplish this goal include being deliberate about when & how we use technology, establishing limits on how much time we spend in front of screens, & giving top priority to pursuits that improve our health. Our mental & physical well-being can be maintained by finding a balance between the benefits of technology & times when we disconnect.

7. How a Digital Detox Can Help in the Long Run

In the long run, your energy, mental clarity, & metabolic health will all benefit from a digital detox practice that you incorporate into your routine. Decreases in screen time over time have been associated with:

Metabolic efficiency, particularly glucose metabolism & fat oxidation, enhanced.

Better sleep, with more rejuvenating cycles of sleep.

Less stress, which helps with hormone balance & inflammation.

Greater physical activity, as less time is spent sitting & more time is spent moving & exercising.

Increased efficiency in both work & playtime as a result of enhanced concentration & output.

Restoring energy, improving metabolic health, & reclaiming vitality can be achieved by regularly incorporating digital detoxes into your routine.

Lifestyle Choices for Long-Term Metabolic Health

Nutritional processing, energy generation, & homeostasis are all aspects of metabolic health that are impacted by various lifestyle choices. Achieving & keeping metabolic health over the long term requires more than just following a strict diet & exercise program; it calls for an all-encompassing strategy for improving one's physical, mental, & emotional health. Weight management, regulating hormones properly, reducing inflammation, & maintaining a balance between energy intake & expenditure are the cornerstones of metabolic health. The foundation of long-term metabolic health is a set of critical lifestyle choices that help achieve these goals. People can better manage the challenges of modern life & lower their risk of metabolic diseases like metabolic syndrome, type 2 diabetes, obesity, & heart disease if they know how to prioritise these habits.

When it comes to lifestyle factors that have a direct impact on metabolic health, nutrition is among the most important. To keep metabolic function at its best, one must eat a diet rich in nutrients & balanced. Proteins, lipids, & carbs are the macronutrients, & vitamins & minerals are the micronutrients, that help keep the metabolism running smoothly in the body. Insulin sensitivity, glucose homeostasis, & adipose tissue formation are all significantly impacted by dietary quality. The antioxidants, fibre, & healthy fats found in plant-based foods like fruits, vegetables, lean meats, whole grains, nuts, & seeds help fuel the body & keep its metabolism running smoothly. By contrast, eating processed foods that are heavy in sugar, bad fats, & additives can throw off your metabolism by making you more insulin resistant, inflammatory, & prone to oxidative stress.

Controlling portion sizes & eating at the right times are two of the most important dietary choices that affect metabolism. Our metabolic health is influenced not only by the foods we eat, but also by the timing & quantity of our meals, according to research. Insulin sensitivity, fat loss, & cellular repair can all be improved through practices like intermittent fasting, in which people eat & then fast for periods of time. Blood sugar levels can be better stabilised throughout the day with smaller, more frequent meals that are nutritionally balanced. This can help reduce the likelihood of insulin spikes & crashes, which can lead to metabolic dysfunction. Overeating increases the risk of metabolic disorders due to increased calorie intake & weight gain; thus, portion control is an additional important component in preventing overeating.

Another pillar of metabolic health over the long run is physical exercise. Consistent physical activity improves insulin sensitivity, increases fat burning, & improves glucose utilisation, all of which have far-reaching effects on metabolic function. How exercise impacts metabolism depends on a number of factors, including the kind, intensity, & frequency of the activity. Strength training activities, like weightlifting or resistance training, aid in the development of lean muscle mass, which is essential for sustaining a higher resting metabolic rate, whereas cardiovascular exercises, like running, cycling, or swimming, enhance cardiovascular health & fat burning. A person's ability to process energy is directly proportional to their lean muscle mass, since muscle tissue burns more calories at rest than fat tissue. The best way to improve metabolic health & avoid weight gain, diabetes, & heart disease is to do strength training in addition to aerobic exercise. Furthermore, stress & chronic inflammation are known to impair metabolism; both can be alleviated through regular physical activity.

If you want to keep your metabolism in good shape, sleep is another important component. A number of metabolic functions, including glucose regulation, fat storage, & appetite control, are directly affected by the amount & quality of sleep. Lack of sleep increases insulin resistance, interferes with hunger hormones like leptin & ghrelin, & makes people crave processed foods that are high in calories & fat. A higher risk of metabolic diseases like type 2 diabetes, increased levels of abdominal fat, & weight gain are all strongly associated with chronic sleep deprivation. Furthermore, energy expenditure is negatively affected by poor sleep, which makes it harder to be physically active the next day. In order to keep metabolic health in check, it is essential to establish good sleep hygiene. This includes things like sticking to a regular sleep schedule, making sure your bedroom is a comfortable place to sleep, & avoiding devices that emit blue light. A healthy metabolism depends on getting the recommended seven to nine hours of sleep every night so the body can repair itself, regulate hormones, & replenish energy reserves.

Managing stress is an important lifestyle component that affects metabolic health, just like proper nutrition, exercise, & sleep. The body's hormonal equilibrium, & the hormone cortisol in particular, are significantly upset by chronic stress. Insulin resistance, fat storage, & an increase hunger for unhealthy foods are all symptoms of metabolic dysfunction, which is often brought on by elevated cortisol levels, which are often the outcome of chronic stress. Adrenal fatigue, caused by the chronic secretion of cortisol, occurs when the adrenal glands are overworked to the point where they cannot generate sufficient quantities of hormones required for the body's regular functioning. A decrease in cortisol levels, an improvement in inflammation levels, & an improvement in metabolic health can be achieved through the practice of stress-reduction techniques like yoga, deep breathing exercises, meditation, & mindfulness. To better manage stress & feel better overall, it's important to take time to relax, unplug from work, & do things that make you happy.

Hydration is an underappreciated component that helps maintain metabolic health. Every cellular process, from energy production & nutrient absorption to waste elimination, depends on the body's water intake. The metabolic rate & the body's capacity to burn fat are both impacted by dehydration. Furthermore, having a proper balance of electrolytes is crucial for proper nerve & muscle function, which in turn contributes to a healthy metabolism. To keep energy levels & metabolic processes running smoothly, it's important to drink enough water throughout the day & eat hydrating foods like fruits & vegetables.

Maintaining good metabolic health over the long run also requires a smoke-free lifestyle. Obesity, insulin resistance, & cardiovascular disease are all associated with metabolic dysfunction, & smoking makes all three more likely. Cigarette smoke contains compounds that boost inflammation, encourage fat storage, & disrupt the body's glucose regulation mechanisms. Metabolic health, disease prevention, & quality of life can all be improved when people stop smoking & don't breathe in secondhand smoke.

Last but not least, maintaining a healthy metabolism requires mindful habits. When we practise mindfulness, we bring awareness to the here & now & make deliberate decisions about everything from food to exercise to how we handle stress. Mindful eating helps us tune into our bodies' signals of fullness & hunger, which in turn helps us avoid overeating & fuel ourselves properly. To avoid becoming too sedentary & falling off the waggon of our fitness goals, it's important to be aware of the types of physical activity we do & to make movement a priority throughout the day. Metabolic function can be indirectly supported by practices like practicing gratitude & positive thinking, which can lower stress levels & improve emotional well-being.

Finally, a well-balanced & efficient energy processing system is the end result of a number of lifestyle choices that contribute to long-term metabolic health. These options include avoiding harmful habits like smoking, getting enough sleep, managing stress, eating a balanced, nutrient-dense diet, & being physically active on a regular basis. In addition to optimising metabolism, reducing the risk of chronic diseases, improving energy levels, & enhancing overall well-being can be achieved by embracing these practices. Realise that maintaining metabolic health isn't about passing a diet or following a fad; it's about developing long-term habits that work in tandem with your body's innate capacities.

Strategies for Optimizing Metabolism

In order to keep a healthy weight, increase energy levels generally, & decrease the likelihood of metabolic diseases, it is crucial to optimise metabolism. Boosting metabolism, improving energy balance, & supporting metabolic health in the long run are all goals we'll aim to achieve in this section. These methods take a more comprehensive approach than just recommending a healthy diet & regular exercise; they take into account the interconnected nature of all the elements that affect metabolism, including but not limited to food, exercise, sleep, stress, & the surrounding environment. Individuals can optimise their metabolism & unlock greater vitality & well-being by adopting a combination of these strategies.

1. Start Eating Foods That Increase Your Metabolism

Optimal metabolism can be achieved in large part through deliberate dietary choices. Consuming nutrient-dense foods can help the body get the antioxidants, vitamins, & minerals it needs to keep its metabolism running smoothly. A faster metabolism can be achieved through the following dietary changes:

Put Protein First: Protein plays an important role in metabolism. A higher thermic effect of food (TEF) is the consequence of digesting protein, as opposed to lipids & carbs, because the digestion of protein uses more energy. Lean meats, eggs, beans, legumes, dairy, & other protein-rich foods can boost post-meal calorie expenditure by as much as 30 percent. Protein also aids in the development & maintenance of muscle mass, an essential component of a healthy metabolism.

Eat More Healthy Fats: To keep your metabolism in good shape, you need to eat more healthy fats like avocados, nuts, seeds, olive oil, fatty fish, & seeds. These fats not only keep you going, but they also play a role in controlling your metabolism through hormones like insulin. One important metabolic process that omega-3 fatty acids seem to enhance is insulin sensitivity.

Select Complex Carbohydrates: Legumes, sweet potatoes, quinoa, & whole grains are examples of complex carbohydrates. Their gradual release of energy helps to stabilise blood sugar levels & provides sustained fuel for the body. Complex carbohydrates, as opposed to the simple carbs found in refined sugars, stabilise blood sugar levels, which in turn reduces the risk of metabolic impairment, cravings, binge eating, & weight gain.

If you want to speed up your metabolism & burn more fat, try adding some of these herbs & spices to your meals. Spices like turmeric & cayenne pepper, for instance, have chemicals in them that make you burn more calories & fat. Caffeine, which is present in both green tea & coffee, is known to increase energy expenditure & so speed up the metabolism.

Keep Yourself Hydrated: The metabolic rate can be drastically reduced if you become dehydrated. In order to absorb nutrients, digest food, & eliminate waste, water is necessary. Because it takes energy to bring cold water to body temperature, drinking it may also temporarily boost metabolism. Aim for 8 to 10 cups of water daily & think about eating more hydrating fruits & vegetables like oranges, watermelon, & cucumbers.

Ensure a Regular Exercise Routine

Among the most effective methods to optimise metabolism is to engage in regular physical activity. Muscle growth, better cardiovascular health, & hormone regulation are just a few of the ways in which exercise raises resting metabolic rate &, by extension, calorie expenditure during exercise. In order to maximise metabolic rate, here are important exercise tactics:

Incorporate Cardiovascular Exercise with Strength Training: Lifting weights & other resistance exercises is an essential part of strength training since it helps you gain lean muscle mass, which in turn raises your metabolic rate. Gaining muscle mass can speed up your metabolism because your muscles burn more calories even when you're not moving around than fat does. Running, cycling, swimming, or dancing are all examples of cardiovascular exercises that can aid in calorie burning, cardiovascular health, & fat loss. To maximise metabolic rate, it is best to do a mix of strength training & cardiovascular exercises.

The acronym HIIT stands for "high-intensity interval training," a type of exercise that uses short bursts of high-intensity exercise followed by shorter recovery periods. Afterburn, the rate at which the body burns calories even after a workout has ended, is enhanced by this form of training. High-intensity interval training (HIIT) is a time-efficient alternative to conventional cardio that can improve metabolic rate, fat burning, & general fitness levels.

In addition to regular exercise, increasing the amount of physical activity you do on a daily basis can also have a major effect on your metabolism. An individual's total energy expenditure can be enhanced by engaging in even the most basic of physical activities—such as walking, taking the stairs, gardening, or simply standing instead of sitting. Aim for 10,000 steps daily for optimal health & think about using a step tracker to keep track of your daily movement.

3. Get the Best Night's Rest for Your Metabolism

A healthy metabolism relies on sleep, which is frequently disregarded despite its critical importance. An increase in insulin resistance, disruption of hunger hormones, &

promotion of fat storage are all detrimental effects of inadequate & poor quality sleep on metabolic function. Boost your metabolism & get a better night's rest by implementing these strategies:

Maintain a Regular Sleep Schedule: The circadian rhythm affects many metabolic processes, so it's important to go to bed & wake up at the same times every day. If you want better sleep & to give your body the time it needs to repair & restore, consistency is key.

The best way to get a good night's rest is to make your bedroom a cool, dark, & peaceful place. To block out distractions, you might want to think about getting some blackout curtains, a white noise machine, or even an eye mask. Improving the quality of sleep you get is another benefit of keeping the room at a comfortable temperature (about 60-67°F, or 15-20°C).

Reduce Your Exposure to Blue Light: The blue light emitted by electronic devices, such as cellphones, laptops, & TVs, can prevent your body from producing the sleep-inducing hormone melatonin. When trying to get a good night's rest, it's best to limit screen time in the hour or so leading up to bedtime & maybe even use blue light filters on your devices.

To help you unwind & get a good night's sleep, try some deep breathing exercises, meditation, or light yoga before bed. Stay away from caffeine & heavy meals in the hours leading up to bedtime; they have a tendency to keep you awake.

Fourth, Reducing Stress to Boost Metabolism

Insulin resistance, weight gain, & the accumulation of abdominal fat are all consequences of elevated cortisol levels, which chronic stress causes. Improving metabolic health requires finding ways to control & lessen stress. Some methods for dealing with stress are as follows:

Activating the parasympathetic nervous system—which promotes relaxation & counteracts the stress response—can be achieved through mindfulness techniques like meditation. Lowering cortisol levels, improving emotional well-being, & supporting metabolic health can be achieved through regular meditation practice.

A great strategy to deal with stress is to engage in physical activity. Regular physical activity lowers cortisol levels, increases the production of endorphins (the "feel-good" hormones), & boosts mood. To effectively manage stress, try to exercise moderately for at least 30 minutes most days.

Read, garden, listen to music, or spend time in nature are all examples of relaxing hobbies that can help you unwind & recharge your batteries. To maintain health & happiness over the long run, it is crucial to do things that make you happy & relax on a regular basis.

5. Remove Environmental Toxins

By interfering with hormone regulation & fostering inflammation, environmental factors like pollutants, toxins, & endocrine-disrupting chemicals (EDCs) can hinder metabolic function. You can optimise your metabolism by reducing your exposure to these harmful substances. Some ways to make the world a better place to live:

Opt for All-Natural Items: Choose non-toxic alternatives to common household products that contain potentially dangerous chemicals such as phthalates, parabens, & bisphenol A (BPA). Metabolic dysfunction & hormonal imbalances have both been associated with these chemicals.

Chlorine, heavy metals, & pesticides are just a few of the potentially metabolically disruptive chemicals found in tap water; to avoid these, it is recommended that you filter your water. Toxins can be removed & water can be made clean & healthy again by installing a high-quality water filter.

Reducing Exposure to Air Pollution: Exposure to polluted air, especially in cities, can harm metabolic health. Spend as little time as possible in polluted areas & think about getting an air purifier for your house if you can.

6. Cultivate Stable Routines for Sustainable Achievement

To be successful in the long run, you need to adopt healthy habits that help your metabolism. Food mindfulness, exercise on a regular basis, stress management, & self-care are all examples of such routines. Furthermore, by lowering stress & encouraging a healthy, balanced lifestyle, positive thinking & emotional wellness can greatly affect metabolism.

Incorporating these practices into your life on a regular basis will set you up for sustained metabolic health, which in turn will bring you more energy, better body composition, & a lower chance of developing chronic diseases. In the end, improving your metabolism isn't a quick fix, but rather a way of life that involves consistently putting your health first.

Nutrition, exercise, sleep, stress management, & environmental factors are all part of the comprehensive approach to metabolic optimisation. A healthier, more energetic life is yours for the taking when you incorporate these tactics into your routine on a regular basis; they will raise your metabolism, boost your energy, & lower your risk of metabolic diseases.

Eating for Energy

The idea behind "eating for energy" is that what we eat has a direct impact on our energy levels & how long we can go without refuelling. At its most fundamental level, energy comes from the macronutrients that our bodies use for fuel: carbohydrates, proteins, & fats. Not only does what we eat affect the efficiency of our metabolism, but it also supplies the raw materials for energy production. Keeping blood sugar levels stable is the first & foremost consideration when fuelling one's body. When we eat a lot of refined sugars or simple carbs, our blood sugar levels will rise quickly & then fall, which can make us feel lethargic, irritated, or exhausted. On the other hand, a steady supply of fuel from foods like complex carbs & healthy fats, which release energy more slowly, helps keep energy levels consistent all day long.

Dietary optimisation for energy requires an emphasis on nutrient-dense, whole foods that sustain metabolic processes. Whole grains, veggies, & legumes are good sources of complex carbs because they take longer to digest, which means that they release glucose into the bloodstream gradually & provide energy over a longer period of time. There is a strong correlation between our digestive health & our energy levels, & these foods are high in fibre, which helps with both. Conversely, sugary snacks, refined grains, & processed foods are good sources of simple carbs, which can trigger fast blood sugar spikes & subsequent drops, which can lead to energy crashes. If you want your body's metabolic processes to stay running smoothly, it's important to eat whole, unprocessed foods that are rich in nutrients. Energy production, muscle function, & nervous system health are all significantly impacted by nutrients like vitamin D, iron, magnesium, & B vitamins.

Protein, like carbohydrates, is crucial for energy production because of the important roles it plays in building & repairing muscles, as well as in immune system function. Protein-rich foods, such as lean meats, eggs, fish, & plant-based alternatives like tofu, beans, & lentils, supply the amino acids needed to maintain energy, especially when you're working out. In addition to preventing the energy dips that come with eating a lot of carbohydrates, protein helps stabilise blood sugar levels by reducing the absorption of glucose. Protein has a somewhat higher thermic effect of food (TEF) than carbs & fats because its digestion uses more energy. This means that eating protein can help you burn more calories & keep your energy levels steady.

When it comes to fuelling the body, healthy fats are also crucial because they offer a steady & long-lasting source of energy. Nuts, avocados, & olive oil are good sources of monounsaturated fats; fatty fish, flaxseeds, & chia seeds are good sources of omega-3 fatty acids, which are essential for hormone regulation, heart health, & brain function. In contrast to carbs & protein, which both provide 4 calories per gramme, fat is an extremely dense source of energy, providing 9 calories per gramme. For tasks that last a long time or necessitate constant focus, fats are a great source of energy. The slow digestion of fats, in contrast to the rapid absorption of simple carbs, allows for a more consistent release of energy throughout the day.

Since water is necessary for practically all metabolic processes, including the production of energy, eating for energy also necessitates proper hydration. When you're dehydrated, your body becomes less efficient at delivering nutrients to cells & eliminating waste products, which can make you feel tired, irritable, & physically slow. For optimal energy generation, electrolyte balance, & hydration, it's best to drink water in sufficient quantities along with electrolyte-rich drinks like mineral water or coconut water. Even moderate dehydration can lower energy levels & impair cognitive function, so it's important to drink plenty of water before, during, & after exercise.

Meal timing is just as important as staying hydrated when it comes to keeping your energy levels consistent. Consuming protein, healthy fats, & complex carbs at regular intervals throughout the day can stave off those pesky energy crashes & hunger pangs that cause people to overeat. If you skip meals, particularly breakfast, you run the risk of experiencing low blood sugar, which can make you feel tired & irritable. To keep from feeling lethargic & sluggish, it's best to keep your meal portions moderate. To keep energy levels optimal & fuel the body consistently, it's better to eat smaller, more balanced meals throughout the day. Instead of sugary cereals or pastries, a well-balanced breakfast with protein & healthy fats can give you steady energy & get your metabolism going for the day.

A nutrient-dense diet, which includes superfoods, can also help you feel more energised. Several foods, including chia seeds, sweet potatoes, blueberries, spinach, & kale, are abundant in minerals, vitamins, & antioxidants that support a healthy metabolism & fight against oxidative stress, which can cause weariness. The caffeine in green tea gives it a subtle energy boost without the jitters of coffee, & the catechins it contains speed up your metabolism, which means you burn more fat & have more stamina. Furthermore, adaptogenic herbs such as rhodiola & ashwagandha can help the body maintain steady energy levels even when things get tough by balancing cortisol levels & providing support when the going gets tough.

Eating mindfully also helps keep energy levels up. To avoid sluggishness caused by overeating & gastrointestinal distress, it is important to pay attention to signals that tell you when you are hungry, eat slowly, & enjoy your food. If you want to get the most energy out of your food, it's best to eat away from electronic devices & other distractions so your body can concentrate on digestion & nutrient absorption.

The last group to think about taking supplements are those with energy-related issues; for example, those who suffer from fatigue due to low iron or B12 levels. Having said that, supplements shouldn't supplant a balanced diet but rather work in tandem with it. To ensure supplements are suitable & helpful for your needs, it is crucial to consult with a healthcare professional before adding them.

In conclusion, eating for energy is more than just filling your stomach; it's about fuelling your body & supporting its metabolic processes with nutrient-dense, balanced meals. People can improve their health, energy levels, & performance in physical activities by eating a varied diet of whole foods that contain complex carbs, lean proteins, healthy fats, & important micronutrients. Eating mindfully, sticking to a regular eating schedule, & staying hydrated all help the body use energy efficiently & avoid the tiredness that comes from eating poorly. Following these steps will not only improve your energy levels, but they will also promote metabolic health in the long run, making it easier for you to maintain peak performance & vigour.

Strategies for Balanced Blood Sugar

The key to good health & plenty of energy is keeping blood sugar levels stable. Fatigue, impatience, cravings, & trouble concentrating are just some of the symptoms that can result from blood sugar fluctuations. A higher risk of developing type 2 diabetes, cardiovascular disease, & obesity can be associated with blood sugar fluctuations that occur frequently over time. Making deliberate decisions about one's food, lifestyle, & surroundings can help stabilize insulin levels & promote metabolic health, which in turn leads to balanced blood sugar. The following are a number of ways to improve your health in the long run, maintain stable energy levels, & control your blood sugar levels.

1. Opt for Foods That Are Whole & Unprocessed

Consuming mostly unprocessed foods is one of the best strategies to control blood sugar levels. Fast spikes in blood sugar, an increase in insulin, & a precipitous drop in energy levels are all symptoms of eating too many processed foods, especially those heavy in refined sugars & simple carbs. Over time, insulin resistance can develop due to the lack of fiber, vitamins, & minerals in processed foods, sugary cereals, white bread, & pastries.

Conversely, the slow energy release of whole foods like vegetables, whole grains, lean meats, & healthy fats aids in keeping blood sugar levels stable. A diet rich in fruits, vegetables, legumes, & whole grains can help keep blood sugar levels steady by reducing the rate at which carbs are digested & absorbed. Fiber also aids in increasing insulin sensitivity, which in turn facilitates better blood sugar management.

Two, Make Use of Lean Proteins & Good Fats

The slow digestion of carbs & the promotion of fullness are two ways in which protein & healthy fats aid in blood sugar stabilization. Blood sugar levels are more stable after eating meals that are well-balanced in protein, fat, & carbs. To avoid dangerous spikes in blood sugar levels following meals, eat protein-rich foods such as lean proteins, eggs, tofu, lentils, & beans.

The absorption of fat-soluble vitamins is aided by healthy fats, which can be found in foods like avocados, nuts, seeds, olive oil, & fatty fish like salmon. These fats also help to reduce inflammation, which is crucial for the proper functioning of insulin. In addition to promoting longer-lasting energy, healthy fats can aid in controlling hunger & preventing overeating by reducing the rate at which sugar enters the bloodstream.

Make Sure Your Meals & Snacks Are Balanced

Eating smaller, more frequent meals that are balanced in carbs, protein, & healthy fats can help maintain blood sugar levels balanced throughout the day. Eating small, frequent meals rather than big, irregular ones helps keep blood sugar levels stable. As an example of a balanced snack, you could have a hard-boiled egg with some veggies or a little handful of almonds with some fruit. Without causing a sugar or carbohydrate crash, these nutrient-dense snacks keep you going all day.

Also, it's best to eat at least three meals a day to keep your blood sugar levels stable; otherwise, you may find yourself craving sugary foods & bingeing later. To get your day started off right & maintain steady blood sugar levels until lunchtime, eat a healthy breakfast that includes protein & good fats.

Fourth, Choose Foods with a Low Glycemic Index (GI)

One way to rank foods based on their carbohydrate content is by looking at their glycemic index (GI). Sugary snacks, potatoes, & white bread all have a high glycemic index (GI), which means they can quickly raise blood sugar levels. Conversely, low GI foods prevent blood sugar spikes & crashes by releasing glucose more slowly into the bloodstream.

Here are some examples of foods with a low GI:

Oats, barley, quinoa, & other whole grains

Leafy greens, cucumbers, & tomatoes are examples of non-starchy veggies.

Legume (black beans, chickpeas, lentils)

Persimmons, berries, apples, & other fruits

One way to keep blood sugar levels steady all day long is to eat more foods with a low glycemic index (GI). Substituting whole grain bread for white bread or sweet potatoes for regular potatoes are two examples of food choices that can drastically affect blood sugar control.

5. Watch Your Serving Sizes

Too much of anything, even nutritious, can throw off your blood sugar levels. When eating foods that are high in carbohydrates, it is particularly crucial to watch portion sizes. Overconsumption of carbs, even from healthy sources like vegetables & whole grains, can overwhelm the body's glucose tolerance.

Half of your plate should be vegetables, quarter should be lean protein, & the remaining quarter should be whole grains or legumes; this is an example of portion control in action. You can control your blood sugar & make sure you're getting all the nutrients you need with this balanced approach.

6. Steer Clear of Sugary & Processed Beverages

One of the leading causes of blood sugar imbalances is drinking sugary drinks like fruit juices, sodas, & energy drinks. Refined sugars abound in these beverages, which are otherwise nutritionally devoid. Their liquid form allows them to swiftly enter the bloodstream & cause a spike in blood sugar levels. While the sugar substitutes in diet drinks won't directly cause a spike in blood sugar, they do have the potential to affect insulin levels & the desire for sugar.

Drinking water, unsweetened tea, or carbonated water can help keep blood sugar levels stable. Make your own naturally flavored drinks at home with herbal infusions or a splash of unsweetened coconut water if you prefer your beverages with a little more sweetness. Another option is to add a slice of lemon or cucumber to water.

7. Get Regular Exercise

One of the best ways to help keep blood sugar levels stable is to exercise. Exercising lowers the risk of insulin resistance by improving insulin sensitivity & increasing glucose absorption by muscles. Consistent physical activity, whether it's walking, cycling, swimming, or strength training, helps maintain metabolic health over the long run & promotes stable glucose control.

Glucose levels after meals can be improved & blood sugar stabilized with even moderate-intensity exercises, like a 30-minute brisk walk. You can maximize your energy levels & glucose metabolism by combining cardiovascular exercise with strength training & flexibility exercises.

8. Make Time to Sleep

A good night's sleep is essential for controlling blood sugar & keeping the body responsive to insulin. Reduced sleep quality is associated with elevated cortisol & insulin resistance, both of which impede the body's ability to control blood sugar levels. A higher risk of developing type 2 diabetes has been associated with elevated blood sugar levels, which in turn are associated with insufficient quality sleep, according to studies.

Get between seven & nine hours of good sleep nightly to help keep blood sugar levels where they should be. To enhance the quality of your sleep, establish a regular sleep schedule, limit screen time in the hours leading up to bed, & make sure your bedroom is comfortable.

9. Keep Stress at Bay

One hormone that has the ability to raise blood sugar levels & exacerbate insulin resistance is cortisol, which can be elevated in response to chronic stress. In addition to exacerbating blood sugar imbalances, stress can cause people to eat poorly, including an increase in cravings for sugary foods. In order to keep blood sugar levels steady, it is crucial to learn to cope with stress.

Think about making time each day for activities that help you relax, like yoga, meditation, deep breathing, or going for a walk in the park. Mindfulness & relaxation practices can aid in regulating blood sugar levels & lowering cortisol.

10. Keep an eye on your glucose levels

It is essential to monitor blood sugar levels on a regular basis for individuals who already have diabetes or prediabetes. Monitoring your blood sugar levels throughout the day with a glucose meter or continuous glucose monitor (CGM) can help you understand the impact of certain foods & lifestyle choices. To maintain healthy blood sugar levels, this information can direct dietary & lifestyle modifications.

Intermittent Fasting & Metabolic Benefits

A lot of people have started to take notice of intermittent fasting (IF) as a way to improve metabolic health, optimize weight management, & boost overall well-being. The focus of intermittent fasting is on when to eat rather than what to eat, in contrast to traditional calorie restriction diets that aim to reduce food intake over a longer period of time. Scientific studies have demonstrated that intermittent fasting can significantly impact many areas of metabolism, including insulin sensitivity & fat-burning capabilities. Intermittent fasting gives many advantages that promote health & vitality in the long run by influencing important metabolic pathways through changing the timing of food consumption.

1. Increased Receptivity to Insulin

Improving insulin sensitivity is one of intermittent fasting's most notable metabolic advantages. By encouraging the uptake of glucose into cells for energy, the pancreatic hormone insulin aids in the regulation of blood sugar levels. But, insulin resistance can set in when insulin levels stay high from overeating, & cells stop responding properly to the hormone. A higher chance of getting type 2 diabetes, more fat storage, & high blood sugar levels are the results.

A decrease in insulin levels & an improvement in insulin sensitivity can be achieved through intermittent fasting, which involves going without food for extended periods of time. Fasting improves glucose metabolism & lowers the risk of insulin resistance; studies reveal that levels of insulin can drop as much as 30 percent in only 24 hours. Maintaining normal blood sugar levels becomes much easier with intermittent fasting, which resets the insulin response by giving the body pauses from continuous insulin secretion.

2. Slimming Down & Enhanced Fat Burning

One more way that intermittent fasting can help you lose weight is by stimulating fat-burning metabolic processes. When you fast, your body uses its glucose stores for energy & begins to rely on fat stores instead. One of the main mechanisms that causes fat loss is lipolysis, the process by which energy is transferred from glucose to fat. Intermittent fasting also aids in the activation of autophagy, a mechanism that eventually leads to fat loss by removing damaged cells (including fat cells).

Intermittent fasting not only enhances fat burning, but it also reduces caloric intake, which contributes to weight loss. Since there is less time for food to enter the body during fasting periods, calorie consumption drops naturally. This causes a calorie deficit, which helps a lot of people lose weight & keep it off. Additionally, research has linked metabolic diseases like diabetes & heart disease to excess visceral fat, which intermittent fasting can help alleviate. This fat is stored around the internal organs.

Thirdly, production of human growth hormone (HGH) has been enhanced.

The hormone known as human growth hormone (HGH) is essential for development, metabolism, & repair. Important for proper metabolic function, it promotes fat loss & muscle gain. The secretion of human growth hormone (HGH) increases during intermittent fasting, particularly during fasting periods, & decreases with age due to natural age-related declines.

Scientific studies have shown that human growth hormone (HGH) levels can be increased by a factor of five after a fast lasting 16 to 24 hours. An increase in human growth hormone aids in fat loss, promotes optimal metabolic function, & helps maintain lean muscle mass. Overall metabolic health is improved by the increased HGH during fasting periods, which also improves exercise performance & muscle recovery.

4. Enhanced Heart Health

By reducing the severity of several major risk factors for cardiovascular disease, intermittent fasting has the potential to improve cardiovascular health. Lower blood pressure, cholesterol, & inflammation are key components in reducing the risk of cardiovascular disease, & regular fasting has been associated to all three. A more favorable ratio of good cholesterol (HDL) to bad cholesterol (LDL) can be achieved through intermittent fasting, which in turn improves lipid metabolism & heart health.

Some of the risk factors for cardiovascular disease, including inflammation & oxidative stress, can be mitigated through intermittent fasting, according to research. Intermittent fasting can help keep your cardiovascular system healthy & lower your risk of developing conditions like high blood pressure, heart attacks, & strokes by lowering inflammation, improving blood lipid profiles, & enhancing fat metabolism.

5. Prolonged Lives & Enhanced Mitochondrial Function

The energy needed for cellular function is produced by mitochondria, which are essentially the cell's powerhouse. Reduced energy production & metabolic dysfunction can result from the natural decline in mitochondrial function that occurs with aging. By increasing the body's production of NAD+, a coenzyme vital for cellular energy production, intermittent fasting has been demonstrated to enhance mitochondrial efficiency & promote mitochondrial biogenesis, the process of creating new mitochondria.

Improving energy levels, metabolism, & cellular repair through enhanced mitochondrial function may lead to an increase in longevity. Experimental evidence from animals suggests that intermittent fasting may increase longevity through enhancing metabolic health, decreasing oxidative stress, & stimulating cellular repair mechanisms. The beneficial effects of intermittent fasting on mitochondrial function offer strong evidence for its potential role in aging & longevity, although further human studies are required to confirm these claims.

6. Cellular Regeneration & Autophagy

When you fast, your cells naturally go into autophagy, a process that eliminates waste, malfunctioning organelles, misfolded proteins, & other damaged or dysfunctional components. In order to keep cells healthy, lower inflammation, & prevent metabolic diseases, autophagy is an essential process.

Particularly when fasting for longer durations, intermittent fasting improves autophagy. Maintaining healthy tissue, optimal metabolic function, & a reduced risk of chronic diseases like cancer, neurodegenerative diseases, & metabolic disorders are all supported by autophagy, which allows the body to repair itself & remove damaged cells.

7. Elucidation of Thought & Cognitive Ability

Cognitive performance, attention, & mental clarity have all been shown to improve with intermittent fasting. Fasting triggers the production of brain-derived neurotrophic factor (BDNF), a protein that promotes brain health, increases learning & memory, & promotes the growth of new neurons. In addition to improving cognitive function & protecting against neurodegenerative diseases like Alzheimer's, fasting periods decrease inflammation & oxidative stress in the brain.

It is believed that the increased production of BDNF & the body's ability to shift to a more efficient energy source—ketones—during prolonged fasting or calorie restriction are responsible for the increased mental alertness & clarity reported by many intermittent fasting practitioners. There is evidence that using ketones, an alternate fuel source for the brain, can enhance cognitive function.

Section 8: Hormonal Control & Metabolic Wellness

A number of important metabolic hormones can be controlled with intermittent fasting. Fasting not only increases levels of human growth hormone, but it also enhances the actions of insulin, the hunger hormone ghrelin, & the satiety hormone leptin. Intermittent fasting promotes optimal hormone release & action, which in turn aids in better regulation of hunger, enhanced fat burning, & more consistent blood sugar levels.

The hormones leptin & ghrelin collaborate to control when we are full. Researchers have discovered that fasting makes people more sensitive to the hormone leptin, which makes it easier for the body to know when it's full & less likely to overeat. At the same time, regulating your ghrelin levels through intermittent fasting will keep you from craving food & experiencing extreme hunger while you're not eating.

A Potent Instrument for Metabolic Wellness: A Conclusion

From better insulin sensitivity & fat burning to improved mitochondrial function & cognitive health, intermittent fasting offers a plethora of metabolic advantages. Intermittent fasting optimizes numerous critical metabolic processes necessary for energy maintenance, weight management, & long-term health by allowing the body to go without food at regular intervals. Intermittent fasting has many potential health benefits, including weight loss, better cardiovascular function, & increased longevity. It is a versatile & effective way to improve metabolic health & live a balanced, healthy life. It is important to be mindful when fasting & pay attention to what your body needs. Make sure that your fasting schedule fits in with your personal health goals & lifestyle.

Meal Timing & Eating Habits to Support Energy

Managing your energy levels throughout the day is greatly influenced by the timing & structure of your meals. Your body's capacity to stabilise blood sugar, regulate hormones, & maintain metabolic function—all of which contribute to sustained energy—is impacted by when & how you eat. Low energy, lethargy, or exhaustion throughout the day is a common problem that many people suffer from due to imbalances in nutrients, poor meal timing, or both. Optimising your nutrition for sustained vitality & better metabolic health is possible when you understand the connection between meal timing, eating patterns, & energy levels.

1. Maintaining Regular Meal Times

Eating at regular intervals is one of the easiest ways to keep your energy levels consistent all day long. Low blood sugar, which can occur when you don't eat for an extended period of time or when you eat too little, makes you cranky, hungry, & irritable. Maintaining steady energy levels & lowering the temptation to overeat later in the day are benefits of eating at regular intervals throughout the day.

The general recommendation is to consume three well-balanced meals per day, with a four- to five-hour gap in between each meal, & one or two little snacks as needed. A typical day in your life might start with breakfast at 7:30 a.m., continue with lunch at 12:30 & dinner at 6:30, with a snack somewhere between 10:30 & 3:30. Your body is able to keep its energy levels & metabolic balance when you adhere to a regular schedule, which helps control your circadian rhythm & promotes better digestion & nutrient absorption.

2. The Significance of Getting a Good Head Start with Breakfast

There is a solid reason why breakfast is considered the most crucial meal of the day. Protein, healthy fats, & fibre make for a well-rounded breakfast that can help you get a jump start on the day, keep your blood sugar levels stable, & keep going strong. Your muscles & brain require a new supply of fuel to get going after a night of fasting because your glycogen stores are depleted.

For long-lasting energy, start your day with a combo of complex carbs (like oats, whole grain toast, or sweet potatoes), protein (like eggs, Greek yoghurt, or nut butter), & healthy fats (like avocados, chia seeds, or almonds). The gradual release of glucose into the bloodstream from these foods prevents energy spikes & crashes.

Breakfast foods heavy in sugar, like sugary cereals or pastries, may give you a short burst of energy, but they quickly wear you down & make you hungry.

3. A Well-Rounded Lunch

Having a healthy lunch is also important for keeping energy levels up. A mid-afternoon slump & reduced productivity can result from skipping lunch or choosing overly processed foods. For sustained energy & less hunger pangs throughout the day, pack a lunch of lean proteins, healthy fats, & complex carbs.

A nutrient-dense lunch that helps maintain steady energy levels is a salad with grilled chicken, avocado, mixed greens, quinoa, & olive oil, for instance. You can slow digestion & get a longer-lasting energy boost by eating meals that are rich in fibre & whole grains. You won't feel as lethargic or exhausted in the afternoon if you don't stuff yourself at lunch.

4. A Rechargeable Snack for Happy Hour

The afternoon is a notoriously low-energy time for many people, particularly between the hours of 2:00 & 4:00. Blood sugar fluctuations, exhaustion, & circadian rhythms are all potential causes of this slump. To keep energy levels up & cut back on later overeating, have a small, well-balanced snack now.

Incorporating protein, healthy fats, & fibre into your afternoon snack is the way to go. An example of this would be a protein smoothie made with spinach, seeds, & nuts, or hummus accompanied by a few carrots. Sugary snacks & caffeine can cause a rapid spike in blood sugar levels, which can be followed by a crash, so it's best to eat a balanced snack instead.

5. The Time & Makeup of Dinner

In the hours leading up to bedtime, eat a smaller, more balanced dinner that still supplies all the nutrients your body needs. Eating supper too late, particularly right before bed, can mess with your digestion & make it hard for you to sleep. To avoid the aches & pains that come from eating too close to bedtime, try to finish your last meal at least three hours before you plan to go to sleep.

At its most ideal, supper should consist of moderate amounts of complex carbs, lean proteins, & veggies. Healthy & filling meals include grilled salmon with roasted veggies or tofu stir-fry with brown rice & a variety of veggies. Eat simple, easily digestible foods that are low in fat & spices to ensure a good night's sleep.

6. Intermittent Fasting & Its Function

Eating in cycles of eating & fasting is called intermittent fasting (IF). While intermittent fasting (IF) isn't for everyone, many people report that fasting for 12–16 hours (e.g., eating nothing between noon & 8 p.m.) helps them control their energy levels, maintain a healthy weight, & boost their metabolism.

Fasting has many benefits, including increasing insulin sensitivity, enhancing cell repair, decreasing inflammation, & allowing the body to use stored fat for energy. If you have trouble controlling your hunger levels or experiencing energy crashes during the day, intermittent fasting may be able to help you stabilise your metabolism & eat less at each meal. During the eating window, though, you should prioritise nutrient-dense foods so that you can reap the most benefits & stay away from nutritional deficiencies.

Section 7: Staying Hydrated & Boosting Energy

Even moderate dehydration can cause headaches, exhaustion, & trouble focussing, so staying properly hydrated is crucial for energy production. Try to stay hydrated all day long, not just between meals. To stay hydrated & promote sustained energy, it's a good idea to drink water frequently & keep a water bottle on hand.

Those who engage in physical activity, in particular, may benefit from supplementing their water intake with herbal teas or electrolyte-rich beverages, such as coconut water. Your body's metabolic processes can be hindered by dehydration, which slows down energy production & makes it less efficient overall. Caffeine can cause energy crashes & sleep disruptions, so it's best to limit your intake.

8. Practices for Mindful Eating

Our digestive & metabolic processes are greatly affected by the food we eat. If you want to improve your digestion & portion control, try eating mindfully—that is, without electronic devices like phones or TV—so you can concentrate on the tastes, textures, & overall experience of your food. Eating slowly & chewing food thoroughly allows your body more time to recognise fullness, which in turn reduces the chances of overeating & post-meal energy slumps.

Better eating habits can be maintained by learning to recognise when you're hungry & not eating when you're bored or stressed. Eating mindfully & appreciatively improves metabolic health & energy levels by making the most of the nutrients in the food.

9. How Energy Is Influenced by Macronutrient Balance

A meal's carbohydrate, protein, & fat content is crucial to your body's energy production & utilisation processes. Carbohydrates are vital for fuelling the brain & muscles because they are the body's principal fuel source. The key is to load up on complex carbs, which provide energy slowly, like those found in fruits, vegetables, & whole grains.

In addition to assisting with blood sugar stabilisation, proteins promote muscle repair & growth. For sustained energy, it's best to eat foods high in protein, like fish, lean meats, eggs, beans, & plant-based proteins. Because they aid digestion & keep you feeling full & energised for longer, healthy fats are essential for sustained energy. Avocados, almonds, seeds, & olive oil are good sources of healthy fats, which aid in metabolism & energy production.

A steady supply of energy from a variety of sources supports metabolism & prevents energy crashes, so it's important to balance these macronutrients in each meal.

10. Planning & Preparing Meals

Meal prepping is a great way to keep to your healthy eating habits & have consistent energy all day long. By making sure you have healthy, well-balanced meals on hand, meal prepping can help you resist the urge to eat junk food or go without meals. Meal prepping allows you to manage portion sizes & incorporates healthy fats, carbs, & protein into your diet in a balanced way.

Maintaining energy levels, supporting metabolic function, & improving overall health all hinge on optimising meal timing & eating habits. You can keep your energy levels up all day long by eating consistently, picking foods that are high in nutrients, & making sure you eat balanced meals. You can improve your capacity to maintain energy levels, which in turn makes you feel energised, alert, & productive, by engaging in practices like mindful eating, drinking plenty of water, & meal prepping. Being mindful of when & what you eat can greatly impact your ability to maintain a healthy metabolism, control your weight, & perform at your best in sports.

Exercise & Metabolic Training

One of the best ways to optimize metabolism, increase energy levels, & support metabolic health in general is to exercise. Being physically active on a regular basis can boost metabolic rate, insulin sensitivity, & nutrient utilization efficiency; the body is a complex system that adjusts to its environment. In addition to the calories you burn during exercise, your metabolism continues to work harder even after you stop moving. This is especially the case when it comes to metabolic training, which entails doing extremely intense exercises with the goal of raising your metabolic rate & encouraging fat burning. Different types of exercise have different effects on metabolic rate, body composition, & energy expenditure; thus, metabolic training is not a cookie-cutter approach.

Metabolic training primarily consists of high-intensity interval training (HIIT) that targets big muscle groups simultaneously. In order to raise heart rate & generate a calorie burn that lasts beyond the workout, this type of training usually consists of short bursts of intense activity followed by short recovery periods. A phenomenon called excess post-exercise oxygen consumption (EPOC) aids in enhancing fat burning, which continues even after the exercise session has ended. The "afterburn" effect describes how your body keeps burning calories even after you've finished a high-intensity metabolic workout. The goal of these exercises is to improve cardiovascular health & maximize energy expenditure by stimulating the aerobic & anaerobic systems simultaneously.

Metabolic training's capacity to target both fat & lean muscle mass is a major advantage. Metabolic training helps burn fat during exercise while simultaneously preserving lean muscle mass & promoting muscle growth, in contrast to steady-state cardio, which mainly burns fat. Resistance exercises, weightlifting, & other strength training components of metabolic workouts are critical for increasing RMR (resting metabolic rate) via muscular stimulation. Increased metabolic rate at rest is a direct result of a higher percentage of lean muscle mass compared to adipose tissue. Metabolic training allows you to burn more calories in less time because it makes use of compound exercises, which work more than one muscle group at a time.

The foundation of metabolic training is high-intensity interval training (HIIT), which helps improve metabolic function & boosts fat loss. High-intensity interval training (HIIT) consists of short, intense bursts of activity followed by shorter rest periods or less strenuous exercise. As an example, a high-intensity interval training (HIIT) routine often consists of 30–45 seconds of maximal effort (e.g., sprinting, jumping squats, burpees, or kettlebell swings) followed by 15–30 seconds of active recovery. The great thing about high-intensity interval training (HIIT) is how quickly you can do it—just 20 to 30 minutes—& yet you'll get a lot of benefits. Studies have demonstrated that high-intensity interval training (HIIT) raises VO2 max, improves fat oxidation, makes the metabolism more flexible, & makes insulin sensitivity higher. The fact that HIIT can be adjusted to suit different fitness levels & objectives makes it suitable for a broad variety of individuals, from novices to elite athletes.

Resistance training, in which you build muscle by lifting weights or utilizing resistance bands, is another effective kind of metabolic training. Although strength training is the most common benefit of resistance training, it also has significant effects on metabolism. Since it takes more energy to maintain muscle than fat, a higher basal metabolic rate (BMR) is associated with a higher amount of muscle mass. To maintain metabolic health as we get older, it is essential to engage in resistance training on a regular basis, as it promotes muscle protein synthesis & aids in the preservation of lean muscle mass. Additionally, it promotes a healthy hormonal balance, which is essential for long-term metabolic function, & it increases bone density & joint stability. Resistance training uses big muscle groups during & after the exercise, which means more calories burned. Some examples of these exercises are squats, deadlifts, lunges, & push-ups.

Cardiovascular health & fat metabolism are two additional areas that metabolic training excels at improving. Aerobic activities, like jogging, cycling, swimming, or fast walking, improve cardiovascular & respiratory efficiency, which boosts oxygen delivery to tissues & aids in fat-burning. Improved blood circulation & a decrease in visceral fat—a dangerous form of fat stored around the organs—are additional benefits of cardiovascular exercise. Aerobic exercise alone isn't enough to boost metabolic rate & body composition; it becomes a potent weapon when mixed with metabolic conditioning exercises & resistance training.

An important indicator of metabolic health is the resting metabolic rate (RMR), which is the quantity of energy that the body expends while at rest. Age, sex, genetics, & body composition are some of the variables that affect RMR. Muscle growth & improved metabolic function are the results of regular exercise, which in turn increases RMR. This is especially true of resistance training & high-intensity workouts. The American College of Sports Medicine actually discovered that after 12 weeks of strength training, participants' RMR increased by 7%. Gaining muscle mass improves metabolic efficiency because, compared to fat, muscle tissue is more metabolically active & hence requires more energy to sustain.

The adaptability of metabolic training is a fascinating feature. People can keep pushing themselves & avoid fitness plateaus thanks to the wide variety of metabolic workouts. If you want to work out in the comfort of your own home or without the need for any special equipment, try some bodyweight exercises like squats, lunges, push-ups, & mountain climbers. If you're looking for a more challenging & varied metabolic training program, you can incorporate resistance bands, kettlebells, dumbbells, or even battle ropes into your routine. Another kind of metabolic conditioning that offers a time-efficient approach to target multiple components of fitness, such as cardiovascular health, strength, & endurance, is circuit training, which incorporates various exercises in a series of stations. A comprehensive approach to metabolic conditioning is achieved by incorporating a variety of movement types into the workout, such as explosive, strength-based, & endurance exercises. This way, the workout targets both the aerobic & anaerobic systems.

Maintaining a regular exercise & metabolism routine is essential. Consistent, long-term effort yields better results than a single high-intensity or resistance training session, although the former can boost calorie burn & metabolic function in the short term. Your body will adjust by using energy more efficiently, burning fat more effectively, & keeping muscle mass as you include metabolic training into your frequent exercise program. A faster metabolism, more energy, better body composition, & a decreased risk of metabolic diseases like type 2 diabetes, obesity, & heart disease are the long-term effects of this.

Remember to take into account your current fitness level, your goals, & your health status when doing metabolic training, just as you would with any other type of exercise. Although high-intensity workouts produce remarkable results, they might not be safe for people who are just starting out or who have preexisting ailments like heart disease or joint pain. Metabolic training at lower intensities, like steady-state cardio or bodyweight exercises, can still be very beneficial for people who are just starting out or who have limitations. To keep pushing the body & improving metabolic health, intensity can be raised gradually as fitness levels rise.

Optimal metabolism, increased energy, & general health can all be achieved through regular exercise & metabolic training. Individuals can increase their energy levels, metabolic rate, fat oxidation, & preservation of lean muscle mass through a regimen that includes cardiovascular exercise, resistance training, & high-intensity workouts. People of all fitness levels can reap the benefits of metabolic training, & it can help improve metabolic health in the long run when added to a balanced exercise program. Exercise can be a potent tool for improving metabolic function, increasing vitality, & living a healthier life if done consistently with the correct balance of intensity & recovery.

Designing a Metabolism-Boosting Workout

In order to design an effective workout that boosts metabolism, one must take into account various components of fitness in order to raise energy expenditure, develop lean muscle, & improve fat-burning mechanisms. In order to promote long-term health & metabolic stimulation, a well-structured exercise program should include cardio, strength training, & high-intensity exercises. For the best results in terms of fat loss, muscle tone, & metabolic flexibility, consider the following when planning your workout:

1. Warm-Up (five to ten minutes)

If you want to avoid injuries, get your muscles ready for intense physical activity, & maximize blood flow, you need to warm up correctly. A good warm-up will get your heart rate up & your muscles ready to go for the workout. Concentrate on kinetic motions like:

One minute of jumping jacks

Do 30 seconds of each of the following: arm circles, shoulder rolls

Squats using only your body weight for one minute

One minute of twisting lunges

Complete 30 seconds of hip circles in each direction.

2. Doing HIIT for fifteen to twenty minutes

When it comes to improving cardiovascular health & speeding up the metabolism, HIIT is a top choice. A brief period of rest or low-intensity exercise follows each set of shorter, more intense bursts of exercise. The increased calorie burn, enhanced fat oxidation, & elevated heart rate are all results of the high-intensity interval training. Using a variety of muscle groups, this HIIT program will help you burn more calories:

High-Intensity Interval Training (HIIT) Program Example:

The full-body explosive movement known as burpees

Climbers of mountains (cardio & core)

Strength & power training with jump squats

Strength training with push-ups

Jump from plank to alternating touching your toes (core & shoulders)

Complete body & power kettlebell swings

With a 30-second break in between sets of four, complete the circuit three or four times. To accommodate different levels of fitness, you can modify the work-to-rest ratio, such as 40 seconds of work & 20 seconds of rest.

3. Strength Training (Twenty to thirty minutes)

If you want to increase your resting metabolic rate (RMR) & gain muscle mass, resistance training is a must. You can increase your metabolic rate, strength, & calorie burn by doing compound exercises, which engage numerous muscle groups all at once. Exercises that target big muscle groups, such as the legs, back, & chest, should be your primary focus.

Complete-Body Resistance Circuit Example:

Performing squats for three sets of ten to twelve repetitions

Squats can be done with the use of bodyweight, barbell, or dumbbells. Squats work the quadriceps, hamstrings, & glutes.

Do three sets of eight to ten repetitions of the deadlift.

The core, glutes, & back are all worked out in a deadlift. Avoid harm by maintaining proper form & keeping your back straight.

three sets of twelve to fifteen push-ups

Using only your bodyweight, you can strengthen your shoulders, chest, & triceps. Perform as directed, adjusting as necessary by getting down on one knee or standing.

3 sets of 8 to 10 repetitions of pull-ups or lat pulldowns

The biceps, shoulders, & back get a good workout with pull-ups & lat pulldowns. Utilize a resistance band or machine to assist with pull-ups if they prove to be too challenging.

Three sets of ten to twelve repetitions of dumbbell lunges on each leg

Improve your balance & coordination while working out your glutes & legs with a good lunge.

Three bundles of twenty twists

Russian twists work the obliques as part of the core. To increase the challenge, you can use a medicine ball or dumbbells.

Rest for 30 to 60 seconds between sets to give your heart a chance to recover. In order to keep your metabolism high & your intensity level constant, this recovery time should be brief.

4. Engage in 20-30 minutes of cardiovascular exercise.

Running, cycling, swimming, or rowing are all forms of cardiovascular exercise that can boost calorie burn, cardiovascular endurance, & fat loss. Maximize the metabolic benefits of cardio by varying the intensity of your workouts.

Typical Exercise Program:

Low-Intensity Cardio (20-30 minutes)

Maintain a steady rate of fat burning by exercising at a moderate intensity (between 60 & 75 percent of your maximum heart rate). Jogging, cycling, or swimming steadily are some possibilities. Aerobic exercise like this promotes fat oxidation & helps burn more calories overall.

Alternating between low- & high-intensity bursts is another option for those who want more intensity & metabolic benefit:

20-minute Tabata-style Cardio

After 10 seconds of rest, do 20 seconds of intense cardio (like a full-out sprint or intense cycling). Finish all eight rounds by cycling backwards & then resting for one minute. As a type of high-intensity interval training (HIIT), tabata training is great for increasing metabolism because of the shorter but more intense intervals.

After that, stretch & cool down for five to ten minutes.

For optimal flexibility & a gradual reduction in heart rate, a cool down is essential. Maintain a static stance for 20 to 30 seconds at a time when stretching. Be sure to warm up & cool down by stretching the muscles you worked.

Stretches for Cooling Down:

A seated or standing hamstring stretch

Standing, bring one foot up to your glutes to stretch your quads.

Stretching the hip flexors (in a lunge position, with the hips pushed forward)

Arm crossed over body is a shoulder stretch.

Extend your arms behind your back to form a chest opener stretch.

In addition to preventing injuries, stretching helps keep muscles flexible & lessens muscle soreness.

6. How Often & How Far Along

Consistency is key if you want to see the best results from your workouts that boost metabolism. Metabolic training should be done at least three to four times per week, with days off for rest or active recovery in between. To keep pushing your body & making progress, it's best to add more volume, intensity, or resistance to your workouts over time. To do this, you can vary the exercises, add sets, use heavier weights, or lengthen the HIIT intervals.

A Weekly Exercise Program Example:

First Day: High-Intensity Interval Training (HIIT) & Total-Body Resistance Exercise

Step 2: Cardio at a Moderate Intensity (Standard Form or Intervals)

Third Day: Relaxation or Physical Recuperation (like Walking or Yoga)

Day 4: Mixed Cardio & Upper Body Strength Training

Fiveth Day: Cardio (High-Intensity Interval Training or Tabata-style routine)

Exercises for the Entire Body & Core Strength on Day 6

The Seventh Day: Do Nothing or Get Moving

Success Hints:

Maintain Consistency: Be consistent if you want to succeed in the long run. Keep to your schedule & push yourself harder as you get in better shape.

To keep yourself hydrated & to aid metabolic processes, drink water before, during, & after exercise.

Eat a variety of macronutrients (protein, lipids, & carbohydrates), micronutrients (small amounts of different nutrients), & fiber to support your exercise program & speed up your metabolism. Fueling your workouts & maximizing recovery are both aided by eating the correct foods at the right times.

A workout that combines cardiovascular exercise, resistance training, & high-intensity interval training will effectively boost metabolism, energy, & fat loss. In the long run, this holistic strategy will boost your metabolic health, body composition, & energy levels.

Incorporating HIIT & Resistance Training

If you want to maximize your metabolism, boost fat loss, & improve overall fitness, an excellent workout regimen to do it with is HIIT & resistance training. When you combine these two effective types of exercise, you get the best of both worlds: better cardiovascular health & stronger muscles. You can increase your calorie burn during & after a workout by alternating between resistance exercises & high-intensity cardiovascular efforts. This will make your muscles work harder & your heart rate rise. A metabolism-boosting regimen that includes both high-intensity interval training (HIIT) & resistance training looks like this:

First, a Fat-Burning Advantage of HIIT & Resistance Training Together: The capacity of HIIT to continue burning fat long after the exercise has ended is one of its most renowned benefits. Your resting metabolic rate (RMR) & calorie expenditure are both enhanced by resistance training, which aids in the development & maintenance of lean muscle mass. A higher resting metabolic rate is associated with increased muscle mass.

Exercises like high-intensity interval training (HIIT) & resistance training don't take up much time at all. You can speed up the process of getting in shape while still getting the advantages of cardiovascular & strength training by combining the two. If you're short on time but still want to get a good workout in, this is for you.

Elevated End-Program Oxygen Consumption (EPOC): When you train with both high-intensity interval training & resistance training, you increase your risk of EPOC, or the "afterburn effect." As it repairs itself after a strenuous exercise, your body keeps burning calories at a high rate. By combining the two forms of exercise, you can increase your EPOC, which means that your calorie burning will be sustained for longer after your workout has ended.

Building & preserving muscle is an important part of a healthy metabolism, & resistance training is a great way to do both. The metabolic rate of muscle tissue is higher than that of fat, so increasing your muscle mass causes you to burn more calories. You can make sure that your body is burning fat & building muscle at the same time by incorporating resistance training into your HIIT sessions.

2. Putting Up a High-Intensity Interval Training & Resistance Training Routine

You can maximize your workout results by alternating between high-intensity interval training (HIIT) & resistance exercises in a circuit or super-set format. The workout should be structured like this:

Effortless Exercise Routine

Whether you're into high-intensity interval training (HIIT) or resistance training, a circuit-style workout is all about moving from one exercise to the next with little to no rest in between. Maintaining a high heart rate during exercise is key to burning as many calories as possible & activating your metabolism to its fullest potential.

Model Exercise Routine (Do 3–4 sets of 30–45 seconds of exercise followed by 15–30 seconds of rest):

HIIT Workout: Squat Jumps

In addition to challenging your cardiovascular system, this explosive movement focuses on strengthening your legs, glutes, & core.

Resistance Training: Deadlifts with Dumbbells

Glutes, hamstrings, & the back get a workout in with this full-body move.

Interval Training with Burpees

This full-body exercise targets the chest, arms, abs, & legs with a high degree of intensity.

Workouts that involve resistance, such as push-ups or dumbbell chest presses, target the upper body.

HIIT Workout: Climbing Stairs

A high-intensity routine that strengthens the abdominal muscles & the heart.

Rowing with dumbbells is a resistance exercise that strengthens the back & biceps.

Strength Training with High Knees

An intense workout that raises the heart rate & tests the lower body.

Strength Training: Squat to Press

Brings the lower body squat & the upper body overhead press together to form a full-body motion.

Rest for one to two minutes after finishing each exercise in the circuit; then, depending on your fitness level, repeat the circuit three to four times.

Format for Super-sets

One compound exercise (multi-joint) & one high-intensity exercise are common examples of the types of exercises used in super-setting, which aim to train different muscle groups simultaneously. You go on to the following pair after finishing one set of each. This approach guarantees that your session includes both cardio & strength training while keeping your heart rate elevated.

Workout Example: Perform four to five sets of each exercise with a 30-second break in between:

Primary set:

Squats with a barbell (10-12 reps)—a resistance exercise

High-Intensity Interval Training: 30 Seconds of Jumps

Secondary set:

Strength Training: Deadlifts (8–10 reps)

High-Intensity Interval Training: Mountain Climbers–30 seconds

Set three:

Strength Training: Shoulder Press with Dumbbells (10-12 reps)

HIIT Workout: 30 Seconds of Burpees

Fourth superset:

Pull-Ups (8-10 reps): A Resistance Exercise

HIIT Workout: High Knees (results in 30 seconds)

You can enhance your aerobic & anaerobic energy systems, which in turn boosts your strength, endurance, & fat-burning capabilities, by alternating between strength-based exercises & high-intensity cardio bursts.

3. Level of Intensity & Advancement

To keep pushing your body to its limits, it is crucial to incorporate progressive overload into your high-intensity interval training (HIIT) & resistance training (RT) routines. To accomplish this, one can:

Step up the intensity by lifting heavier weights or extending the time between high-intensity interval training (HIIT) sets (from 30 to 45 seconds, for example).

Exercising Differently: In order to avoid reaching a fitness plateau, it is recommended to switch up the exercises you do every few weeks. For example, instead of doing kettlebell swings or barbell squats, try goblet squats or jump squats.

Cutting Down on Downtime: To maintain an elevated heart rate & maximize the metabolic benefits, gradually decrease the rest period between exercises or rounds.

4. A Weeklong Exercise Program Example

To make sure you're working out every part of your body, try mixing high-intensity interval training (HIIT) with resistance training. Give me an example of a weekly schedule:

First Day: Total-Body Circuit Workout (HIIT + Resistance)

Day 2: Engage in some light stretching, yoga, or walking to aid in your recovery.

On the third day, you'll focus on your lower body via HIIT & lower body resistance training.

On Day 4, you'll focus on strengthening your upper body through resistance training & high-intensity interval training (HIIT).

Day 5: Highly-Optimal Cardio or Full-Body Circuit (Optional for Elite Athletes)

For Day 6, you can either relax or get some exercise by swimming, cycling, or light jogging.

Day 7: Cardio with Core Work (High-Intensity Interval Training & Static Cardio)

5. A Diet to Supplement Your High-Intensity Interval Training & Resistance Training programme

Proper nutrition, in addition to exercise, will fuel your metabolism-boosting workouts. To help you achieve your fitness goals, a healthy diet should consist of:

Protein: Consume lean protein sources like chicken, turkey, tofu, eggs, or legumes frequently after resistance training to help repair & build muscle tissue.

Carbohydrates: Consume enough carbs, particularly before high-intensity interval training (HIIT), since they are the body's principal source of energy. Instead of simple carbs, go for complex carbs like oats, brown rice, sweet potatoes, & whole grains.

Nuts, avocados, & olive oil are good sources of healthy fats that can help regulate your hormone production & energy levels.

Be sure to drink lots of water before, during, & after your workouts to stay properly hydrated. This will help with performance, recovery, & metabolic function.

6. Recuperation & Rest

Rest & recovery are crucial after high-intensity interval training (HIIT) & resistance training. In order to maximize metabolic function, restore muscle fibers, & fill up glycogen stores, your body requires rest. Make sure you're getting seven to nine hours of sleep nightly & that you give your muscles a full day of rest every week.

Rest & Recovery: The Importance of Active Recovery

Although they are just as important as the workouts themselves, rest & recovery are frequently disregarded when planning an effective exercise program. In particular, active recovery has emerged as an essential component for maximizing fitness gains, promoting metabolic health, & avoiding injuries. In contrast to passive rest, which entails lying down & doing nothing, active recovery promotes low-intensity movement to increase blood flow, decrease muscle pain, & hasten recovery after strenuous physical activity. Better long-term results, improved performance, & an enhanced sense of well-being can be yours when you include active recovery into your fitness regimen. This way, your body can recover while still reaping the benefits of movement. A wide variety of light aerobic exercises, such as walking, swimming, or cycling, as well as mobility & flexibility-focused stretching routines, yoga, & Pilates, are all part of an active recovery program. This kind of recuperation lessens the likelihood of overuse injuries, enhances mobility, & can even keep calories burned even when you don't exercise as vigorously. In addition to easing stress & giving a break from high-intensity exercise, it can aid in mental recovery. Beyond its obvious physiological benefits, active recovery can regulate metabolic processes like hormone production & cellular repair—two of the most important factors in achieving & maintaining a healthy metabolic rate & optimal energy balance. The body repairs microtears in muscles, restores glycogen levels, & clears metabolic waste products like lactic acid that accumulate during intense physical activity during periods of active recovery. A well-rounded fitness regimen must include active recovery because it helps reduce inflammation, improves sleep, & keeps the cardiovascular system active. The body adjusts to the demands of past workouts by getting stronger, more efficient, & more prepared to deal with future physical challenges as you recover. In addition, it allows for contemplation & awareness, which helps people pay attention to their bodies & modify their workouts appropriately. In order to improve performance & maintain metabolic health & vitality in the long run, it is essential to understand the value of rest, & active recovery in particular. Individuals can improve their health in the long run, train more effectively, & minimize the likelihood of injury by including active recovery into their comprehensive fitness program. Longevity in fitness & general health are ensured by striking a balance between intense workouts & active recovery. This allows the body to continue progressing without the negative effects of overtraining.

Sleep Hygiene & Stress Reduction Techniques

Better metabolic health, faster recovery, & general wellness can be yours with the help of a well-designed sleep environment & the application of effective stress reduction strategies. The body's physiological processes, including energy levels, cognition, hormone balance, & immune system function, are regulated by a combination of good sleep hygiene & stress management. Implementing habits that promote restorative sleep is part of good sleep hygiene, while learning to reduce stress is an important part of managing the chronic stress that can interfere with sleep, slow down metabolic processes, & even cause some health problems. When taken as a whole, these habits have far-reaching consequences for metabolic health, impacting not only nutrient processing but also fat burning & muscle maintenance. A regular & soothing nighttime routine is the first step in good sleep hygiene because it sends a message to the body that it is time to wind down & transition from the awake state needed during the day to the relaxed state needed for a good night's sleep. Establishing a regular bedtime & wake-up time, keeping the bedroom dark, peaceful, & cool, & avoiding stimulating activities or substances like caffeine, alcohol, or strenuous exercise in the hours leading up to bedtime are all part of this routine. The body's circadian rhythm is improved by being exposed to natural light during the day, particularly in the morning. This makes it easier to fall asleep at night & stay awake during the day. For optimal mental & metabolic health, stress management is just as important as good sleep hygiene. Hormonal imbalances caused by chronic stress, including cortisol, adrenaline, & insulin, have a direct impact on energy regulation & metabolism, & chronic stress also disrupts sleep patterns. In response to stress, the body goes into "fight or flight" mode, which raises blood pressure & heart rate & triggers the secretion of cortisol, the principal stress hormone. Although short-term stress may be tolerated, long-term stress has far-reaching effects on metabolic health, making one more prone to insulin resistance, obesity, cardiovascular disease, diabetes, & other chronic conditions. Some ways to deal with stress include practising mindfulness, deep breathing, yoga, meditation, & progressive muscle relaxation. Initiating the parasympathetic nervous system through these methods aids in relaxation, decreases cortisol levels, & brings metabolic balance back into the body. Also, getting regular exercise, especially mindful activities like yoga or tai chi, can help you relax, sleep better, & maintain a healthy metabolism. In addition to facilitating better decision-making & a more balanced lifestyle, getting enough sleep & managing stress are associated with enhanced mental clarity, emotional regulation, & focus. In addition, reducing stress & getting enough sleep both aid the body's recovery processes following exercise by repairing damaged muscles, restocking glycogen stores, & maintaining a healthy balance of hormones like testosterone & growth hormone. A more robust feeling of energy, improved metabolic efficiency, & longer-term success with weight management are the end results. Every part of health can benefit from a comprehensive strategy that combines effective stress reduction techniques with good sleep hygiene practices. Managing stress & getting enough sleep are two cornerstones that should be prioritized by anyone seeking to maximize their energy & metabolism. An individual's physical performance, metabolic balance, & long-term health can be improved by creating a soothing sleep environment & implementing stress reduction & management strategies.

Creating a Sleep-Enhancing Environment

If you want to improve your metabolic health, mental clarity, emotional regulation, & general well-being—& get a good night's sleep—one of the best things you can do is make your bedroom a sleep-enhancing environment. Designing the bedroom such that it encourages relaxation & supports the body's natural sleep cycle is important because it is a place where one should go to rest. Light, noise, temperature, & the quality of one's sleeping surface are just a few of the many aspects of one's sleep environment that should be carefully considered in order to maximize the likelihood of a restful night's sleep & a feeling of well-rested upon awakening. Managing the amount of light entering a room is one of the most important things you can do to make it easier to sleep. The internal clock that regulates the sleep-wake cycle can be thrown off by prolonged exposure to light, especially blue light emitted by screens. By interfering with the secretion of the sleep-regulating hormone melatonin, this disturbance, which is referred to as circadian misalignment, can hinder metabolic health, delay the start of sleep, & decrease the quality of sleep. Limiting exposure to bright or blue light in the evening, especially from electronic devices like smartphones, tablets, or televisions, is essential for creating an ideal environment. Keeping bedroom lighting at low levels promotes the production of melatonin, which helps with the transition into sleep, & using warm light bulbs or installing dim lighting in the bedroom can signal to the body that it is time to wind down. The opposite is true: being outside in the sunshine first thing in the morning can help you get a better night's sleep by regulating your circadian rhythm. On top of that, when you're trying to get some shut-eye, your bedroom should be pitch black. To accomplish this, one can use blackout drapes, blinds, or even an eye mask to shield one's eyes from light, which the body uses to regulate its circadian rhythm. As soon as it gets dark, the brain receives the signal to start making melatonin, which in turn promotes deeper sleep. Managing noise levels is another crucial component of a sleep-enhancing environment. For a good night's sleep, you need to be in a peaceful environment free of distractions.

Even mild noise can interfere with your natural sleep cycle, especially during the more rejuvenating stages. The deeper stages of the sleep cycle are essential for physical recovery, hormone regulation, & memory consolidation; however, environmental noises like traffic, household sounds, or appliance hums can disrupt this process. If you're having trouble sleeping due to excessive noise, try utilizing earplugs, a white noise generator, or even just a fan. For a more restful night's sleep, try using white noise, which is a steady stream of calming sounds that can mask more disruptive sounds. Maintaining a comfortable temperature while sleeping is another important consideration. A room that is excessively hot or cold can disrupt the body's natural process of lowering its core temperature in preparation for sleep. Because cooler temperatures help the body's thermoregulation, sleeping better is associated with keeping the bedroom at a temperature between 60 & 67 degrees Fahrenheit (15 & 20 degrees Celsius). If you have trouble falling or staying asleep because the room is too hot, try turning down the thermostat a few notches. Alternatively, if the room is too chilly, it might hinder the body's ability to unwind & enter deeper stages of sleep. Bedding & sleep surfaces are also important components of a conducive sleep environment. To ensure correct spinal alignment & a state of neutral repose, choose a mattress & pillows that provide both comfort & support. Discomfort from an unevenly firm or soft mattress, or from pillows that don't offer adequate support, can interrupt a good night's sleep & make it difficult to relax. Finding the ideal sleeping arrangement for one's own needs requires trying out various mattresses, pillow kinds, & bedding materials. Another thing that can help you stay at a comfortable temperature all night long is to use bedding made of breathable, soft materials like linen or cotton. Improving one's sleep hygiene is aided by maintaining a tidy & uncluttered environment. Clutter in the bedroom is associated with increased stress & anxiety, which in turn makes it harder to relax & unwind. An organized bedroom with few distractions is a great place to relax & get a good night's sleep. In order to train your body to associate the bedroom with relaxation & rejuvenation, you should use it mainly for sleeping & relaxing, not for work or entertainment. Additional ways to improve the sleeping environment include the use of aesthetic components like calming colors, gentle textures, & calming aromas. Decorate your bedroom with soothing colors like gentle blues, greens, & earth tones to help you unwind & relax. Also, you can help your nervous system relax & get a better night's sleep by using aromatherapy diffusers or essential oils scented with sandalwood, chamomile, or lavender. Research has demonstrated that aromatherapy can alleviate anxiety, slow the heart rate, & enhance the quality of sleep. Adding plants to your bedroom can have its advantages as well. Some plants, like jasmine or lavender, have calming effects that can help you get a better night's sleep. Consideration of fresh air circulation is an additional aspect. To enhance the sleep environment by lowering carbon dioxide buildup & promoting better oxygen exchange, it is recommended to open a window for ventilation if at all feasible. A room with good ventilation can aid in body relaxation, allowing for a more restorative night's sleep. Although having a comfortable bedroom is essential for getting a good night's rest, sticking to a regular sleep schedule is even more crucial. Making your bedroom a relaxing place to sleep is important, but so are developing routines that let your body know it's time to wind down. Maintaining a regular bedtime & wake time—even on weekends—helps normalize the circadian rhythm, which in turn makes it easier to fall asleep & wake up without artificial stimulation. Reading, soaking in a warm bath, or doing deep breathing exercises are all great ways to wind down before bed, which can help your body & mind get ready for a good night's sleep by easing tension & preparing you for a peaceful night's sleep. In the hours preceding bedtime, stay away from things that can disrupt sleep, such as heavy meals, caffeine, alcohol, or strenuous physical activity. This will help create an environment that is conducive to sleep. Individuals can improve their metabolic health, energy levels, & mental & physical performance throughout the day by focusing on creating a conducive sleep environment & implementing consistent sleep habits. This will lead to deeper & better sleep.

Effective Stress-Relief Practices

Managing the physiological & psychological effects of stress is crucial for maintaining good health, a healthy metabolism, & general well-being. Many medical problems, including anxiety, depression, metabolic dysfunction, heart disease, & autoimmune disorders, can be triggered by prolonged exposure to stress. While the body's stress response is meant to keep us safe in dangerous situations, it can become overactive & cause issues like chronic inflammation, hormone imbalances, & insomnia if activated too often or for too long. Consequently, to lessen the impact of these drawbacks, it is crucial to build stress-reduction techniques into everyday life. Research has demonstrated that mindfulness meditation can lower cortisol levels, improve emotional regulation, & increase cognitive focus, making it one of the most effective stress-relief practices. Mindfulness is the practice of nonjudgmental attention to the here & now; it helps people overcome stress by breaking the habit of worrying or overthinking. Meditation practices that cultivate awareness of the present moment, such as counting breaths or performing body scans, have a calming effect on the central nervous system, increase relaxation, & strengthen emotional resilience. Research has shown that regular practice of even brief periods of mindfulness can have a profound effect on one's mood, level of self-awareness, & reduction of stress. To activate the parasympathetic nervous system, which is responsible for the body's relaxation response, deep breathing is an effective stress-relief technique that entails deliberately slowing the breath & engaging the diaphragm. A simple yet effective way to reduce acute stress & calm the body is to practice deep breathing exercises like diaphragmatic breathing, box breathing, or 4-7-8 breathing. Incorporating these exercises into your routine can help alleviate stress by lowering your heart rate, blood pressure, & promoting a state of calm & relaxation. Practicing these breathing techniques can bring a sense of calm & stability, which is particularly helpful when dealing with stressful or anxious situations. Another great method for reducing stress & tension is progressive muscle relaxation (PMR). Participants in progressive muscle relaxation (PMR) work their way up from the feet to the head, systematically tensing & releasing each group of muscles. Deep relaxation is the result of this practice's ability to heighten awareness of the body, alleviate pent-up tension, & activate the parasympathetic nervous system. Individuals can learn to manage stress before it gets out of hand by developing a heightened awareness of their bodies' tension points. Because it induces a state of complete relaxation throughout the body, PMR is especially useful for people who suffer from physical manifestations of stress, like headaches, muscular tension, or gastrointestinal problems. Tai chi & yoga are mind-body practices that integrate breathing exercises, physical postures, & meditation to enhance health, alleviate tension, & increase flexibility. Slow, controlled movements are a hallmark of both tai chi & yoga, which in turn promotes awareness of one's breath & body, which in turn heightens the relaxation response & soothes the neurological system. These practices not only help you relax, but they also boost your physical health by making you more balanced, better at your posture, & with better blood flow. For profound relaxation, try a restorative or yin yoga practice. These styles emphasize passive stretching for long durations, which helps the body release tension & regain balance. An integrative method for alleviating stress, yoga is even more effective when combined with meditation or mindfulness practices. An additional great tool for stress management is exercise, especially aerobic & strength-training workouts. Exercising releases endorphins, which are like little elevators for your mood; they lift your spirits & make you feel good about yourself. So, when you work out, you may say goodbye to anxiety & depression. In addition to lowering cortisol levels, exercise boosts BDNF production, a protein that helps the brain stay healthy & resilient in the face of stress. Moderate exercise, like walking, cycling, or swimming, on a regular basis has long-term advantages, including better cardiovascular health, better sleep, & stabilized blood sugar levels. Intense workouts may provide short-term stress relief, but moderate exercise builds resilience & balance in the body. Even if you find vigorous exercise too much to handle when you're stressed, low-impact exercises like walking, light swimming, or even stretching can help you relax & be more mindful. Another straightforward method that works wonders for dealing with stress & releasing pent-up emotions is keeping a journal. Putting pen to paper allows one to express themselves emotionally, which in turn helps one to better understand & cope with their challenges. Those who have trouble controlling their thoughts & feelings can find that keeping a journal helps them do just that by allowing them to write down their ideas in an organized & external format. Journaling, whether with free-writing or guided prompts, allows people to reflect on their emotions & recognize patterns that might be causing stress. This, in turn, gives them the power to make positive changes in their lives. People can learn more about their stress responses & triggers by keeping a regular journal, which also helps with mindfulness & self-awareness. Retaining positive relationships with others is another effective method for reducing stress. Because it allows for the possibility of emotional validation, connection, & reassurance, social support is essential in lowering stress levels. One way to deal with stress is to talk to someone, whether it's a friend, family member, or therapist. This can help with processing emotions, getting a different view, & feeling less alone. Volunteering, attending community events, spending time with loved ones, & other positive social activities can all contribute to a sense of well-being & alleviate feelings of loneliness & anxiety. Toxic or negative relationships can worsen stress & damage mental health, so it's crucial to make sure that your social interactions are supportive & nurturing instead. Research also shows that being outside, whether that's strolling through a park, going for a hike in the woods, or just sitting on the beach, can help to relax both the mind & the body. Being in nature makes people feel better emotionally, physically, & mentally. It also decreases stress hormones & makes them feel more relaxed. Taking a break from technology & spending time in nature is a great way to reset your brain, which in turn can help you feel less stressed & more focused. Managing one's time well & establishing limits are other essential components of stress management. Work, family, & social responsibilities can quickly become too much for people in today's fast-paced society. Preventing burnout & excessive stress can be as simple as learning to say "no" & setting priorities. Task batching & the Pomodoro Technique are two examples of time management strategies that can help people concentrate, reduce stress, & make more room in their schedules for leisure activities & self-care. One way to achieve a better work-life balance is to learn to delegate responsibilities, cut out the fluff, & set attainable goals. Lastly, cultivating an optimistic outlook & making an effort to be grateful can greatly enhance one's ability to handle stress. One way to alleviate stress & cultivate optimism is to concentrate on the positive aspects of life rather than dwelling on problems. One way to change one's perspective on stress & make it more manageable & less overwhelming is to keep a thankfulness notebook or to take moments throughout the day to reflect on things for which one is grateful. In conclusion, there is no one best way to alleviate stress; rather, it is a combination of approaches, including but not limited to physical exercise, journaling, social connection, & mindfulness & relaxation exercises. A person's metabolic health, resilience to stress, & general health can all be improved by making these practices a regular part of their lives. Participating in stress-reduction activities on a regular basis has multiple health benefits, including enhanced emotional & mental well-being, improved sleep quality, hormonal balance, & a stronger immune system. Individuals can lessen stress's negative effects, promote metabolic health, & develop a stronger sense of vitality & balance by creating a stress-management regimen that fits their specific needs & way of life.

Meditation, Breathing, & Mindfulness for Energy

It is often disregarded how meditation, breathing exercises, & mindfulness practices affect energy levels & metabolism, despite their long-established reputation as potent tools for improving mental clarity, emotional wellness, & general health. The foundational principle of these practices is to assist individuals in reestablishing harmony between their physical, emotional, & mental selves, which in turn promotes a state of sustained energy & vitality. The capacity to quiet the mind, which is a common source of mental & physical fatigue, is central to meditation's role in boosting energy. Regular meditation practice activates the parasympathetic nervous system, which counteracts the stress-related "fight or flight" response by promoting the body's "rest & digest" functions. This change in the autonomic nervous system helps reduce levels of cortisol & other stress hormones, which, when continuously elevated, can reduce energy levels by affecting metabolic function, causing fatigue, & interfering with sleep patterns. You can improve your mood & energy levels by meditating, which acts as a mental reset, enabling you to break free from cycles of stress, anxiety, or burnout. Through the practice of meditation, one can achieve inner calm & harmony, which in turn restores energy to the body. Mindfulness meditation is among the best ways to increase energy through meditation. Practicing mindfulness entails bringing one's whole attention to the here & now, nonjudgmental observation of internal experiences (such as thoughts & emotions), & increased sensitivity to external bodily sensations. The ability to concentrate & focus is improved through this practice, leading to a more energised & effective mind. Reduced mental fatigue & improved cognitive function can lead to a greater sense of clarity & mental energy through mindfulness meditation. This practice trains the brain to focus on the present moment rather than dwelling on past events or future uncertainties. Negative emotions, like stress, anxiety, or frustration, can drain energy, but mindfulness meditation can help regulate these feelings. Slowly but surely, those who make mindfulness a habit may find that it improves their overall well-being, allowing them to face life's inevitable ups & downs with poise & determination rather than exhaustion. An additional effective strategy to boost energy levels is to practice targeted breathing exercises in conjunction with meditation. Controlled breathing, often known as breathwork, is a method of altering one's physiological state through deliberate regulation of breathing. Diaphragmatic breathing, often called abdominal or deep breathing, is a popular breathwork technique for increasing energy. One way to practice this technique is to breathe deeply into the diaphragm. As you inhale, expand your belly & let it fall naturally as you exhale. The parasympathetic nervous system is activated by diaphragmatic breathing, which in turn lowers blood pressure, slows the heart rate, & promotes relaxation. Additionally, it boosts oxygen delivery to cells, which in turn increases energy reserves. Reducing anxiety symptoms, increasing lung capacity, & fostering a calm, energized state of mind are all possible outcomes of regular deep breathing practice. The 4-7-8 breathing method is another breathwork technique that is great for increasing energy levels. Participants in this method take four deep breaths in, hold them for seven, & then release them for eight. By calming the muscles & triggering the parasympathetic nervous system, this exercise has dual benefits: reducing stress & increasing energy levels. The regularity of breathing induces a state of awareness known as mindfulness, in which one pays closer attention to one's physical self & the here & now. Consequently, the 4-7-8 technique is commonly employed to alleviate stress, anxiety, or exhaustion, offering a rapid infusion of energy when one is emotionally or physically drained. Square breathing, also known as box breathing, is another easy way to boost your energy. Participants in this technique inhale for four counts, hold for four more, exhale for four, & repeat the process. Through activating the parasympathetic nervous system, which promotes relaxation & mental clarity, this breathing pattern improves oxygenation of the body, heightens concentration, & decreases stress. When you're feeling overwhelmed or exhausted, practicing box breathing regularly can help you concentrate better, calm your nerves, & reenergize. Integrating breathing exercises with mindfulness meditation can provide a more complete picture of how to boost energy. They work hand in hand to assist people in developing a profound awareness & presence, which in turn can alleviate mental noise & fatigue. Restoring energy, reducing mental fatigue, & improving overall well-being can be achieved through the practice of both meditation & breathwork. When done consistently, the synergistic effects of these practices increase, allowing you to go through the day with boundless energy. A person's metabolic function can be optimized through the practice of meditation & breathing techniques. Chronic stress can impair metabolic processes including digestion, nutrient absorption, & hormone regulation; reducing its negative effects requires slowing down the breath & calming the nervous system. Researchers have discovered that cortisol, a hormone that can affect insulin sensitivity, fat storage, & blood sugar regulation, is secreted more frequently in people who are under chronic stress. A healthy metabolism allows the body to produce & use energy more efficiently, & mindfulness &

breathwork can help reduce stress. Improved sleep quality has a direct effect on metabolic health & energy levels; practices like meditation & mindful breathing can help with this. Fatigue, impaired cognitive function, & hormonal imbalances affecting energy regulation, cravings, & appetite can result from inadequate or poor sleep. People can help their bodies wind down for a better night's sleep by meditating & practicing breathing exercises in the hours leading up to bedtime. Consistent meditation & breathwork can help you get deeper sleep, which is necessary for recharging your batteries, regulating your metabolism, & healing your body. Incorporating practices like mindfulness, deep breathing, & meditation into one's daily routines can help one become more emotionally resilient. These methods aid people in controlling their reactions to difficult situations, which in turn lessens the emotional toll that negative thought patterns can take. Reducing emotional reactivity—a major energy drain—is possible when people learn to observe their emotions without judgment or attachment. A person may feel mentally & physically drained after dealing with intense emotions like wrath, frustration, or anxiety. By establishing emotional distance through meditation & mindfulness practices, people are better able to respond to challenging situations with composure & clarity. A more positive emotional state & more energy can result from practicing emotional detachment over time. Practicing mindfulness, deep breathing, & meditation on a regular basis has physical health benefits as well. Muscle tension decreases, blood circulation improves, & oxygen delivery to tissues is enhanced when the body is relaxed. The body is able to recover from stress & physical exertion with the help of this relaxation response, which helps conserve energy. As a result, this recuperation boosts general vigor & performance in physical activities & everyday life. A state of relaxation allows the body to work more efficiently, allowing it to save energy for more meaningful pursuits while decreasing the amount of effort needed for mundane chores. A comprehensive strategy for increasing energy, addressing the psychological & physiological causes of energy loss, can be achieved through the practice of meditation, breathwork, & mindfulness. Breathwork increases oxygen delivery & relaxation, meditation helps reestablish emotional & mental balance, & mindfulness increases awareness & presence in the here & now. When combined, these practices form an effective framework for maximizing health, lowering stress, & increasing energy. People can strengthen their mental clarity, physical health, & emotional equilibrium by making these practices a part of their everyday lives. Improve your metabolism, increase your vitality, & improve your quality of life with the help of meditation, breathing exercises, & mindfulness practices. These can be utilized either as a short-term energy restorer or as part of a longer-term plan for health & wellness.

www.ingramcontent.com/pod-product-compliance
Lightning Source LLC
Chambersburg PA
CBHW051048250726

48656CB00001B/204